Essential Medicines Management for Mental Health Nurses

Deborah Robertson

Mc Graw Hill Education Open University Press

Open University Press
McGraw-Hill Education
8th Floor
338 Euston Road
London
NW1 3BH

email: enquiries@openup.co.uk
world wide web: www.openup.co.uk

and Two Penn Plaza, New York, NY 10121-2289, USA

First published 2016

A catalogue record of this book is available from the British Library

ISBN-13: 978-0-33-526398-1
ISBN-10: 0-33-526398-4
eISBN: 978-0-33-526399-88

Library of Congress Cataloging-in-Publication Data
CIP data applied for

Typeset by Aptara, Inc.
Printed and bound by CPI Group (UK) Ltd, Croydon, CR0 4YY

Praise for this book

"A knowledge and understanding of medicines and medication management is a fundamental aspect of the role of the mental health nurse. The author succeeds in her aim of providing of both a basic knowledge of the subject area, and an understanding of how the principles of psychopharmacology and medicines management are applied to clinical practice and the role of the nurse.

The book has an excellent structure, each chapter beginning with clear learning objectives, and ending with a summary of key learning points; multiple choice questions, and a case study, where relevant. The text is written in an accessible style; specific chapters, for example, chapter 5 "Anatomy and physiology of the brain", having clear diagrams that facilitate the reader's ability to understand both basic physiology, and the principles of neurotransmission, etc. The role of the therapeutic alliance is helpfully acknowledged when promoting adherence and concordance, whilst the key medications prescribed for the specified disorders, and the associated psychopharmacology, are clearly described.

I would consider the publication as being essential reading for any undergraduate mental health nurse; the text also being a valuable learning resource in the development of curriculum content."
Mark James, Senior Lecturer in Community Mental Health Nursing, University of South Wales, UK

"I'm delighted to recommend this new, welcome and accessible resource: an excellent book with much to offer student and registered mental health nurses and nurse educators, in promoting safe and effective practice in medicines management. With an easy to understand style, Deborah Robertson provides a helpful overview of the legal and professional context, a practical introduction to undertaking drug calculations, and considers the complex issues around practical strategies for optimising adherence and patient outcomes. Complementing recommended non-pharmacological interventions for well-known mental health disorders, this book offers a refreshing perspective and special focus upon pharmacological treatment options, clearly explaining the use of specific medications, their main modes of action, effects and side effects, and recommendations for monitoring outcomes.

In particular, this book offers the reader a very good grounding in understanding the pathophysiology and pharmacological treatment of mental health disorders, providing materials and highlighting further resources for use when working with the patient or service user, whether providing education, involving them in decision-making about medication taking, or actively monitoring outcomes. Another valuable feature is that the reader is encouraged to consolidate their learning through a series of reflective case studies that focus upon recognising need and treatment planning, and end of chapter multiple choice and numeracy questions."
John Butler Senior Lecturer in Mental Health, University of Central Lancashire, UK

"This book comprehensively addresses all the major psychotropic drugs a mental health nurse will encounter when undertaking medicines interventions. Each mental health diagnosis is explored and the related prescribed medicines covered in depth. I would recommend this book for use as a core text book in undergraduate studies, registered nurses who want to increase their knowledge base and for non-medical prescribing students as a baseline source to learn about the psychopharmacology of drugs they will prescribe."

Steve Hemingway, Senior Lecturer in Mental Health, The University of Huddersfield, UK

I would like to thank my husband and son for their support and patience during the writing of this book; without their encouragement I would have enjoyed this journey much less. This book is for Alex.

Brief table of contents

Detailed table of contents

About the author

Deborah joined the faculty of Health and Social Care at the University of Chester in 2004, where she is currently employed as a senior lecturer in the department of Public Health & Wellbeing.

She is a registered general nurse (RGN) but also holds a BSc (Hons) and PhD in pharmacology. Her PhD was on the subject of lymphatic vessels in sepsis, but her post-doctoral fellowship work was in the area of mental health with a specific focus, over her 3-year funded work, on stress and depression.

She is currently the programme leader for the non-medical prescribing course, where she uses her expertise in pharmacology, but also leads on and contributes to other modules within the faculty including research in community practice, psychopharmacology and perspectives in pharmacology. She also inputs into the undergraduate nursing teaching and curriculum.

Her current research interests involve e-learning and the delivery of the non-medical prescribing course.

Deborah is married and has a teenage son.

About the contributor

Dr Alexander Robertson is a general practitioner with an interest in mental health disorders. He has contributed to the discussion around the clinical and non-pharmacological management of the conditions in Chapters 6, 7, 8, 9, 10 and 13.

List of abbreviations

AMHP	approved mental health practitioner
BNF	British National Formulary
BNFC	British National Formulary for Children
CBT	cognitive–behavioural therapy
CG	Clinical Guideline (from NICE)
CQC	Care Quality Commission
CTO	community treatment order
DVLA	Driving and Vehicle Licensing Agency
ECG	electrocardiogram
GABA	gamma-aminobutyric acid
GAD	generalized anxiety disorder
GP	general practitioner
HADS	Hospital Anxiety and Depression Scale
HbA_{1c}	haemoglobin A_{1c}
ICD-10	International Classification of Disease, 10th revision
IM	intramuscular
IV	intravenous
MAOI	monoamine oxidase inhibitor
MDT	multidisciplinary team
MHRA	Medicines & Healthcare Products Regulatory Agency
MHT	mental health tribunal
NARI	noradrenaline reuptake inhibitor
NHS	National Health Service
NICE	National Institute for Health and Care Excellence
NMC	Nursing and Midwifery Council
OCD	obsessive–compulsive disorder
PHQ	Patient Health Questionnaire
POM	prescription-only medicines
PTSD	post-traumatic stress disorder
RC	Responsible Clinician
SC	subcutaneous
SI	standard international (international system of units)
SSRI	selective serotonin reuptake inhibitor
TCA	tricyclic antidepressant
WHO	World Health Organization

Introduction

Pharmacology and medicines management is something that my student nurses tell me all the time, is very important to them. They also tell me that the subject of psychopharmacology is daunting and often find the textbooks dedicated to it 'overwhelming', 'difficult to understand', 'over our heads', 'not real life' and 'expensive'. I don't know that I can say this book solves all of those issues, but I know that writing this book, with students (and nurses in general) in mind, has made me very aware of those issues when deciding how to lay out chapters and to display information. Nurses need to understand pharmacology and medicines management, yes, no question. But they also need to know how to apply this knowledge to the patients in their care. This book links theory to practice in every chapter and helps nurses transfer their learning from the page to the practice situation.

Nurses often say they wish there was more pharmacology taught at undergraduate level, but as an educator I understand the pressures of a nursing programme and the importance of all the other subjects taught. However, as a nurse and pharmacologist I see and understand their point. As educators we instil the importance of pharmacological knowledge and teach the basics of pharmacology to give students the 'building blocks' of knowledge. But each student and their experience in practice is very different, so knowing where to find and how to use information is still one of the best skills we can teach. Combine this with enthusiasm for a subject and a lifelong learner is born.

Learning about medicines as a nurse is fundamental to a major component of the role they will play (medicines management) and the care they will deliver, so motivating students to learn about drugs in an easy, accessible and applicable format is essential. This book is written with that purpose in mind. There is a proverb that sums this up well for me: 'Give a man a fish, and you feed him for a day; show him how to catch fish, and you feed him for a lifetime.'

This book does not give you all the snapshots of pharmacological information for you to pick and eat for the day you want. It gives you basic knowledge, clinical understanding and the tools to find and apply information that will have you 'fishing' for pharmacological knowledge every day for the rest of your career.

An introduction to mental health and medicines management

1

Chapter contents

Before you begin...
Learning objectives
Introduction
What is mental health and mental illness?
The prevalence of mental health disorders

The mental health nurse
Key learning points
Multiple choice questions
Recommended website
Recommended further reading

Before you begin...

Medicines management is an important area of nursing and healthcare practice that all practising professionals can and should be involved in. Mental health nursing is no exception, and the mental health nurse should have a good grasp of pharmacology and medication use to be a safe and effective practitioner. Although patient management in mental health does not always involve medication, for many patients you will come across medication is the mainstay of their treatment. What the

medication does, how it works, how to give it and what to look out for are all important areas of knowledge that all mental health nurses must have. This book aims to help the mental health nurse, at whatever stage of their career, to develop and maintain that knowledge.

Now we have set the scene, read on. This first chapter introduces mental health and illness and the mental health nurse's role in caring for people suffering with mental health problems.

Learning objectives

After reading this chapter you will have gained knowledge around:

- What is meant by the terms mental health and mental illness.
- The range of mental health disorders.
- The prevalence of mental health disorders.
- The role of the mental health nurse.

Introduction

Mental health and wellbeing affects all of us, from childhood, through adolescence into adulthood, and into old age. It often involves how we perceive ourselves and how we think and feel about things. It can affect our ability to cope with situations and our relationships with others. It is not more or less important than physical health – just different! That does not mean that mental and physical health are not linked (often they are); just that we must address issues in both spheres of life as they arise.

We all have times where we feel low or down, sad or frightened, stressed or anxious. This is 'normal' in our life, but if these things are not transient and go on to develop into a more serious problem then we may be described as having a disorder of our mental health. We as healthcare professionals often hear people say 'I am depressed' and sometimes this is inaccurate, as that person is not suffering from a clinically diagnosed depression but is experiencing a normal low in their life. But as lifestyles and jobs change, and stress is very much part of 21st century life, it is essential that we recognize the importance of mental health and crucial that we can diagnose disorders of our mental health that require treatment and intervention.

What is mental health and mental illness?

When asked about 'what is mental health and illness?' many people will be able to tell you that mental illnesses are depression and schizophrenia. As a mental health nurse you will come across many people requiring care due to these disorders, but it is important to realize there are a wide range of mental health conditions and we will explore some of these in this book. They can be categorized for ease as seen in Table 1.1.

Mental health disorders are formally categorized in the *International Statistical Classification of Diseases and Related Health Problems 10th Revision* (ICD-10) World Health Organization (WHO) Version for 2016. This gives a more detailed classification of diseases and is the reference point for many health professionals.

Although stress is not classified as a mental health disorder it is recognized that stress can be

Table 1.1 Categories of mental health disorder

Category	Condition
Anxiety disorders	GAD (Generalized anxiety disorder)
	PTSD (Post-traumatic stress disorder)
	Social phobia
	Panic disorder
	OCD (Obsessive–compulsive disorder)
Mixed anxiety and depression	Mixed anxiety and depression
Depressive disorders	Unipolar depression
	Bipolar affective disorder
Psychotic disorders	Schizophrenia
	Psychotic disorders
Dementias	Alzheimer's disease
	Lewy body dementia
	Multi-infarct dementia
Substance misuse	Drug addiction
	Alcohol addiction
Eating disorders	Anorexia
	Bulimia

a major contributory factor in the development of, in particular, anxiety and depression. Stress of events and places is linked with social phobia, post-traumatic stress disorder (PTSD) and recurrent depression. It is a factor taken into consideration in the assessment of patients presenting with a mental health problem.

The aim of treating a mental health disorder is to promote recovery and return the patient to a functional capacity. This can be achieved using talking therapies, medication or a combination of both. An approach focused on promoting the patient's recovery has the nurse and other mental health professionals working with the patient to support them in living their lives in a fulfilling and significant way. This can promote social inclusion and avoid the stigma and isolation that can be attributed to those suffering from mental ill health. Sometimes recovery does not mean absence of symptoms and many people with mental health conditions do have ongoing symptoms, but it is more about helping them accept and manage those symptoms to allow them to get on with their daily life.

Many medications are available for use in mental health conditions and we will be looking at which drugs help which disorders in the specific chapters to come. The general names of classes of drugs we use are shown in Table 1.2.

Table 1.2   Drugs used in mental health disorders

Disorder categories	Drug classes used
Anxiety disorders	Anxiolytics
	Hypnotics
	Beta blockers
Depressive disorders including mixed anxiety and depression and bipolar affective disorder	Antidepressants
	Anxiolytics
	Hypnotics
	Mood stabilizer
Psychotic disorders	Neuroleptics
	Antipsychotics
	Anxiolytics
Dementias	Acetlycholinesterase inhibitors
	Antidepressants
	Hypnotics
	Anxiolytics
Substance misuse	Replacement therapies
	Aversion therapies
	Symptom management
Eating disorders	Antidepressants
	Anxiolytics

The prevalence of mental health disorders

Mental health disorders are fairly prevalent within the UK with one in four British adults experiencing at least one diagnosable mental health problem

in any one year, and one in six experiencing this at any given time (*Adult Psychiatric Morbidity Report, 2007*, McManus et al. 2009). This means that at any given time around one quarter of the UK population is experiencing a mental health problem. This gives us an idea of the scale of mental health problems that the National Health Service (NHS) is dealing with year in, year out. The most commonly diagnosed of those is mixed anxiety and depression, according to the *Adult Psychiatric Morbidity Report, 2007*. These figures are for the population as a whole, but if we look into the data further there are some revealing facts.

The gender split is favoured towards more women than men receiving treatment suggesting either women are more likely to have a mental health disorder *or* they are more likely to seek treatment for it. This is interesting enough, but if we look at rates of suicide the gender balance shifts with men being three times more likely to die by suicide than women. Alarmingly we see that around one tenth of the child population is diagnosed with a mental health problem. It is not just the young and adults, however, that mental health disorders affect as around one in five older people have a diagnosis of a depressive condition. Mental health problems are common within the UK prison population with the report showing that only one in ten prisoners at that time had *no* mental health disorder. Mental health nurses commonly work in our prison services for this very reason.

It is notable that mental health problems make up a significant proportion of 'ill health' and indeed are a leading cause of workplace sickness and absence. These lost work days place a considerable financial burden upon employers and the economy in general. The timely and appropriate recognition of mental health conditions can help to reduce severity of conditions and allows for prompt intervention to promote recovery.

The mental health nurse

Mental health nurses provide care to people of all ages, who are currently in the throes of, or are at risk of developing, mental health problems. This does not mean that as a mental health nurse you will only treat mental health problems as you will provide care and treatment to meet people's physical, psychological, social, mental and spiritual care needs. This is similar to all fields of nursing practice. In fact it is important to consider physical health as we know that mental health can have an impact on physical health and vice versa. But in general in mental health nursing your focus will be on psychological issues.

The role of the mental health nurse is not simply a hospital based one. They work with patients (or clients as they are often described) in a multitude of settings. This includes hospital work but also they have roles in community settings, day services, crisis interventions, forensic settings and very often in the patient's or client's home. The role often comprises a variety of skills with empathy and interpersonal skills being key. They can perform general care duties or offer specialist interventions around talking therapy, group activities, recovery work and medicines management. Their role is embedded in the concept of 'recovery'. Recovery in mental health does not mean a patient being 'cured' of their condition but is more related to the management of their mental health and a feeling of empowerment or being in control of their life, even when suffering from a mental health disorder. The recovery model of care is a holistic one where the actions and involvement of the mental health nurse are fundamentally focused on the person rather than the condition. All of the above make nursing in mental health a very challenging yet rewarding career path.

Key learning points

Mental health disorders

▶ There are a variety of conditions categorized as mental health disorders.
▶ The most prevalent mental health disorder is mixed anxiety and depression.
▶ Medications can be used to aid recovery in mental health with or without talking therapies.

The mental health nurse

▶ The mental health nurse provides care in a variety of settings to people of all ages, with – or at risk of – mental health problems.

Multiple choice questions

Try answering these multiple choice questions to test what you have learned from reading this chapter. You can check your answers on page 149.

1 **Depression can be described as**

   a) Unipolar and multipolar
   b) Multipolar and oligopolar
   c) Oligopolar and bipolar
   d) Unipolar and bipolar

→

←

2 Neuroleptic medication is used for

a) Psychosis
b) Neurosis
c) Epilepsy
d) Parkinson's disease

3 What is the most common serious mental health condition?

a) Psychosis
b) Depression
c) Anxiety
d) Mixed anxiety and depression

4 Mental health disorders can occur

a) Only in adults
b) Only in developed countries
c) To anyone at any time
d) Only in response to stress

5 Physical health conditions can impact on mental health. True or false?

a) True
b) False
c) Only in terminal illness
d) Only if pain is present

6 How many people in the UK are thought to have suffered from a mental health disorder according to statistics from 2007?

a) 1 in 100
b) 1 in 10
c) 1 in 4
d) Everyone

7 Stress can be said to be

a) A mental health condition
b) Something only anxious people get
c) Only a problem in adults
d) Contributory to many mental health disorders

8 Mental health conditions are most prevalent in

a) Children
b) Women

→

←

    c) Men

    d) Elderly people

9 Work absence due to depression is

    a) An increase on economic burden

    b) A decrease on economic burden

    c) Minimal compared with back pain

    d) Around 5 days per person per year

10 Mental health nurses work increasingly with

    a) Depressed patients

    b) Anxious patients

    c) Drug and alcohol problems

    d) A wide range of mental health disorders

Recommended website

The Mental Health Foundation: http://www.mentalhealth.org.uk/

Recommended further reading

McManus, S., Meltzer, H., Brugha, T., Bebbington, P. and Jenkins, R. (2009) *Adult Psychiatric Morbidity Report, 2007*. London: The NHS Information Centre for Health and Social Care. Available at: http://www.hscic.gov.uk/pubs/psychiatricmorbidity07 (accessed 19 February 2016).

World Health Organization (WHO) (2016) *International Statistical Classification of Diseases and Related Health Problems 10th Revision (ICD-10) – WHO Version for 2016*. Available at http://apps.who.int/classifications/icd10/browse/2016/en (accessed 19 February 2016).

Legal and ethical aspects

2

Chapter contents

Learning objectives
Introduction
Legislation in the field of mental health
Accountability and responsibility
Consent and capacity
Ethical considerations

The role of the nurse
Professional guidelines and standards for practice
Key learning points
Multiple choice questions
Case study
Recommended further reading

Learning objectives

After reading this chapter you will have gained knowledge around:

- The legislation relating to mental health.
- The legislation relating to medicines and prescribing.
- The issue of consent and the capacity to give or withhold consent.
- Your accountability, responsibility and role in medicines management.
- The role of ethics in mental healthcare.
- The place of professional guidelines and standards in relation to mental health nursing.

Introduction

It is important that the nurse involved in the care, treatment and assessment of patients with a mental health disorder has a good awareness of the legal, ethical and professional aspects in the area of mental health. There is a wealth of legislation surrounding this and it can be quite daunting to think of all of these laws and acts. In addition to the law there are professional frameworks we must work within and moral and ethical codes to which we must adhere. This chapter will summarize and discuss the main laws surrounding the care and treatment of the person with a mental health disorder and explore the professional and ethical aspects relating to the law.

Legislation in the field of mental health

The Mental Health Act 1983 (amended)

This is the main primary legislation governing the formal detention and care of mentally disordered people in hospital and the community in England and Wales. The old 1959 Mental Health Act was

Table 2.1   The Mental Health Act – parts and provision

Part of Act and title	Areas covered
Part 1 – Application of Act	Mental disorder
Part 2 – Compulsory admission to hospital and guardianship	Procedures for admission Treatment Guardianship Duration of stay Aftercare
Part 3 – Patients concerned in criminal proceedings or under sentence	Remands to hospital Restriction orders Detention and transfer
Part 4 – Consent to treatment	Plans of treatment Consent Emergency treatment
Part 5 – Mental health review tribunals	Constitution Application and references Discharge
Part 6 – Removal and return of patients within the UK	Covers Channel Islands, Isle of Man, Scotland & Northern Ireland law and transport Removal of aliens Patients absent without leave
Part 7 – Management of property and affairs of patients	Court involvement Judges powers Procedure
Part 8 – Miscellaneous functions of local authorities and the Secretary of State	Approved Mental Health Professionals (AMHP) Visiting Aftercare Secretary of State functions
Part 9 – Offences	Forgery or falsehood Ill treatment Obstruction
Part 10 – Miscellaneous and supplementary	As title states

repeated in 1983 and the present Act came into force the same year. The Act was amended again by the Mental Health (Patients in the Community) Act 1995. A further amendment came in 2007 and this is the current version of the Act used in practice. This Act is concerned with the procedures, safeguards and circumstances in which someone suffering from a mental health disorder can be detained for treatment if necessary without their consent to protect them or the public at large from harm.

The Act is split into parts with additional schedules. The areas covered by each part are separated into sections. These are outlined in Table 2.1.

Important sections for nurses to consider

Section 135(1) Power of entry and removal:

- If it is reasonably suspected that a person is suffering from a mental disorder and is unable to care for themselves, an approved mental health practitioner (AMHP) can seek a warrant from a magistrates' court. This warrant authorizes the police, accompanied by an AMHP and/ or a doctor to enter locked premises.
- A patient, if removed, can then be taken to a place of safety (usually the hospital but not always) and can be kept there for up to 72 hours for assessment.
- Treatment can only be given with the patient's consent or in an emergency.
- Following assessment a patient may be discharged, admitted to hospital informally or further detained under the Mental Health Act.

Section 136 Mentally disordered persons found in public places:

- This section authorizes a police officer who finds a person who appears to be suffering from a mental disorder, in a place to which the public have access, to remove them to a place of safety.
- A person removed to a place of safety can be detained there for up to 72 hours to be examined by a doctor and interviewed by an AMHP.

- Treatment can only be given with the patient's consent.
- The person can then be released from hospital, agree to a voluntary admission or be further detained under the Mental Health Act.

Section 5(4) Nurse's holding power:

- Allows a nurse of the prescribed class (usually a qualified mental health nurse) to detain an informal or voluntary patient who is already being treated for a mental disorder for up to six hours if they deem that it is necessary for their health and safety that they do not leave the hospital.
- The holding power lapses on arrival of a doctor or appropriate clinician who can detain the patient under section 5(2), see below.
- Treatment can only be given with the patient's consent or in an emergency.
- If the patient leaves the hospital or ward area without permission, they can be returned if found within the six-hour time period.
- The patient can agree to stay informally or be detained under section 5(2)

Section 5(2) Doctor's holding power:

- This provides for the detention of an informal or voluntary patient who is already being treated for a mental disorder for 72 hours by a doctor, if they deem that it is necessary for their health and safety that they do not leave the hospital.
- Only one medical recommendation is required.
- Treatment can only be given with the patient's consent or in an emergency.
- If the patient leaves the hospital or ward area without permission, they can be returned if found within the 72-hour time period.
- The Responsible Clinician (RC) can discharge the patient at any time within the 72-hour time period if it is appropriate to do so.
- After this the patient may return to informal status if:
  - an assessment for Section 2 or 3 (see below for detail) is carried out and it is decided

that no further section is necessary; for example, the patient may change their mind and decide to remain in hospital voluntarily;

■ an AMHP may decide an application is not necessary even though two doctors have made medical recommendations for further detention under Section 2 or 3.

■ Possible outcomes:
  ■ the patient agrees to stay on an informal basis;
  ■ the patient is further detained under Section 2 or 3.

Compulsory detention orders

Parts 2 and 3 of the Mental Health Act deal with compulsory admission and detention in hospital for up to 28 days under Section 2 for assessment, or assessment followed by treatment. It is not renewable and if continued detention is required it may be followed by a Section 3.

It requires two medical recommendations and one AMHP application. Consultation with the nearest relative is not required.

■ The patient's consent to treatment should be sought; however, treatment may be given against the patient's wishes.

■ The RC may grant leave of absence if it is deemed appropriate to do so.

■ If the patient leaves the hospital without permission, they can be returned within the 28-day period.

■ The RC can discharge the patient at any time within the 28 days.

■ There are other discharge possibilities:
  ■ application by nearest relative;
  ■ hospital manager's review;
  ■ mental health tribunal (MHT);
  ■ if further detention is required the patient then needs to be detained under Section 3.

Section 3 allows compulsory detention for treatment for up to six months, and is renewable for six months in the first instances and then for periods of one year. It requires two medical recommendations and one application by an AMHP. Consultation with the nearest relative is also required.

■ Treatment can be given for the first three months without the patient's consent. After three months the RC has to get the patient's consent or request a Second Opinion Doctor from the Care Quality Commission (CQC) in order for the treatment to continue.

■ Leave of absence can be granted by the RC for any time limit for up to the expiry of the section.

■ If the patient leaves the hospital without permission, they can be returned to hospital.

■ The RC can discharge the patient at any time during the six months.

■ There are other discharge possibilities:
  ■ nearest relative appeal;
  ■ hospital manager's review;
  ■ MHT.

Mental health tribunals

■ The First Tier Tribunal Service is an independent judicial body established under the Tribunals, Courts and Enforcement Act 2007 (MHT). It has the power to decide whether patients should continue to be detained.

■ It is independent and acts just like a 'mobile court'.

■ Members of the tribunals are drawn from members of the legal profession, doctors and lay people. The legal member will chair the Hearing. Restricted cases are chaired by a judge.

■ Hearings are held with all participants present.

The MHT has the power to:

■ Discharge patients from hospital.

■ Decide on delayed discharge, conditional discharge or transfer to another hospital.

■ Adjourn the Hearing if further information is necessary.

■ Recommend leave of absence or community treatment orders (CTO).

■ Reconvene if recommendations are not complied with.

The MHT requires medical, nursing and social circumstances reports before the Hearing. Prior to the Hearing the medical member will visit the patient and look at the notes. Reports should be produced several weeks before a Section 3 hearing for distribution to tribunal members, the patient and the patient's legal representative. The patient receives copies of all reports. Any information that a team feel should be withheld from the patient should be submitted separately and clearly marked as confidential.

The Care Quality Commission

The CQC replaced the Mental Health Act Commission under the amended Mental Health Act. They monitor, inspect and regulate health and social care services and publish their findings in the public domain. Their responsibilities with regard to mental healthcare include:

- Reviewing the ope ration of the Mental Health Act and the way in which powers of detention are exercised.
- Monitoring the Consent to Treatment provisions of the Act to ensure patients' rights are maintained.
- Carrying out official visits to hospitals to talk to patients and professionals and inspect documentation.
- Monitoring the use of the Code of Practice.
- Reporting biennially to Parliament.
- Providing second opinion approved doctors for Consent to Treatment.
- Receiving complaints from detained patients.
- Monitoring deaths of detained patients.

Any person authorized by the CQC has the right of access to detained patients and their records.

Although members of the CQC generally give notice of their intention to visit, they can make unannounced visits and it is an offence to refuse an authorized person access to patients or their records.

Assessment and treatment under the Mental Health Act is covered by National Institute for Health and Care Excellence (NICE) guidance; Clinical guideline (CG) 136 *Service User Experience in Adult Mental Health Services* (2012) has a section specifically devoted to best practice and care and guidance to healthcare professionals who may be involved in the process.

The Mental Capacity Act 2005

The Mental Capacity Act of 2005 is set out to protect and empower people who may be, either temporarily or permanently, unable to make a decision for themselves. This can be around decisions in day-to-day living as well as healthcare assessment and treatment. It is in three parts and has additional schedules as shown in Table 2.2.

The Mental Capacity Act tells us as healthcare professionals that we should assume an adult individual has the capacity to reach their own decisions until such time as is proven otherwise through a capacity assessment. This will be further discussed in this chapter under consent and capacity.

The Medicines Act 1968

It is important that you are aware of this and its purposes; it will be discussed in more detail in Chapter 11.

Table 2.2 The Mental Capacity Act – parts and provision

Part of Act and title	Areas covered
Part 1 – Persons who lack capacity	Information around capacity and assessment Power of attorney Court powers Advanced decisions and healthcare treatment
Part 2 –The Court of Protection and the Public Guardian	The Court of Protection Powers, practice and procedures Fees and costs The Public Guardian and their function
Part 3 – Miscellaneous and general	As title states

- The act controls the production and supply of medicinal products.
- Its main purpose is to protect the public from harm, i.e. to ensure as far as possible that medicinal products are safe and effective.
- It identifies practitioners that have the authority to prescribe.
- It also restricts the availability of medicines by classifying them as:
  - general sales list: GSL;
  - pharmacy medicines: P;
  - prescription-only medicines: POM.

Other legislation

Nurses must also be familiar with other legislation regarding care of patients with a mental health disorder including:

- The Human Rights Act 1998.
- The Equality Act 2010.
- The Mental Health (Discrimination) Act 2013.
- The Code of Conduct of the Nursing and Midwifery Council (NMC).

Accountability and responsibility

All healthcare professionals owe a duty of care to the patients and clients they work with. This comes under the heading of accountability and responsibility with regard to our NMC Code of Conduct. This changes dependent on whether or not you are a student or registered practitioner and is well outlined by the NMC. Let us look at the concepts of responsibility and accountability in turn.

Responsibility is an ethical or ideological theory that an entity, whether it is a government, corporation, organization or individual, has a duty to society at large. As a nurse we hold a responsibility to our patients, their carers and relatives, our colleagues, the NHS and the NMC and society at large to carry out care to an expected standard and with compassion and competence. It is also there to ensure that the care we give is in adherence to the law, ethical standards, and local/national/international norms.

Accountability is a concept in ethics with several meanings. It is often used synonymously with such concepts as:

- responsibility;
- answerability;
- enforcement;
- blameworthiness;
- liability.

It is often associated with the expectation of account-giving. As an aspect of clinical governance, it has been central to discussions related to problems in both the public and private worlds. For example, if a nurse did not give a prescribed medicine they would have to give a rationale (account) for *why* they had omitted the medication and why this was in the best interests of the patient or what they did after not giving the drug.

Professionals such as nurses, doctors and others involved in healthcare can be called on at any time to account for and justify their actions and omissions. They would be judged against criteria that are held up to be the normal standards of their profession usually detailed in the code of conduct they must adhere to. These standards may also be set out in the areas of healthcare law. Accountability is the acknowledgment and assumption of responsibility for the actions, omissions and consequences of such actions and omissions of the healthcare professional in the conduct of their normal practice. This is usually set by job descriptions, banding or role responsibilities outlined in employment contracts. Indeed, the NMC Code of Conduct (2015) reminds us that we are accountable for our actions in all areas of our practice.

Consent and capacity

Consent is an important part of healthcare law and an ethical principle that nurses are expected to adhere to. Consent by a patient to receive (or to decline) treatment is the principle that they must give their permission *before* any type of medical treatment, procedure or examination is undertaken. This can and should only be done after an appropriate explanation and sufficient information is given by a healthcare professional responsible for or involved in the care of that patient.

Consent can be given in the following ways.

- Verbal – for example, by saying they are happy to accept treatment, a procedure or an examination after explanation and information is given.
- Written – for example, by signing a consent form for surgery after explanation and information is given.
- Implied– for example, when asked if they can have their blood pressure taken the patient holds out their arm to show they know what is to be done to them. This is a very passive form of consent and does not assume capacity to consent is present so must be used with caution in circumstances where the patient's capacity to consent is impaired or uncertain.

For consent to be deemed as valid consent in law the patient must have given it freely and must have not been coerced in any way. Valid consent is only so if it is informed consent. The patient has to have full knowledge of the actions and consequences that they are consenting to. They should also be informed of the consequences if they do not consent to treatment, for example, how their condition may progress if they do not start a medication deemed essential by a healthcare professional. Finally, for valid consent, the person giving consent must be capable of giving that consent, meaning not just that they have been given the information required to make the decision but that they understand that information and can use it to decide to give or withhold permission to proceed.

Capacity is the term we use for capability to consent. This should be assessed by the healthcare professional before or at the time consent is sought. The following issues would be relevant when assessing capacity:

- age – children and some adolescents may lack capacity due to immaturity;
- mental state – mental impairment or disturbance due to mental health issues;
- learning disability;
- loss of consciousness;
- intoxication due to alcohol or drugs.

As you can see someone can lack the capacity to consent for many reasons but we shall discuss the issues around mental disturbance or impairment here. For the issues of a person of young age, see Chapter 12 on mental health medication in children and adolescents. To be deemed unable to consent due to lack of capacity, the person is assessed by someone trained and experienced in assessing capacity and who is involved in the patient's care at the time consent is required. They must determine the following points.

- Can the person understand the information that is being given to them?
- Can the person remember the information given to them?
- Can they use the information they have been given to reach a decision?
- Can they communicate this decision to the person taking consent?

If a person is deemed to have capacity at the time of assessment then their decision to give or withhold consent to treatment must be respected. Patients with capacity should be free to make these decisions without any form of undue pressure or any element of coercion by the healthcare professional seeking the consent.

If a person is deemed not to have capacity at the time of assessment then their decision to give or withhold consent to treatment needs to be carefully looked at by the healthcare professional seeking the consent. They may then choose to continue with the proposed treatment in the best interests of their patient. This must be documented at the time. They may decide to withhold treatment if it is safe to do so until the person regains the capacity to consent if this is possible.

Treatment can go ahead where necessary without consent for a person without capacity to consent if:

- waiting until they do have capacity is unsafe;
- the patient has been involved in the decision as much as possible; and
- the healthcare professional has tried to gain the views of relatives or carers where appropriate.

For more information you may wish to review the contents of the Mental Capacity Act 2005.

Ethical considerations

Ethical considerations are an important aspect of care for any patient but are especially necessary when dealing with people who have a mental health disorder. Many healthcare professionals work through an ethical decision-making framework when faced with ethical matters, such as the one outlined below (Jameton 1984).

Ethical decision-making framework

- Identify the problem.
- Gather additional information.
- Identify all the options open to the decision-maker.
- Think the situation through.
- Make the decision.
- Act and assess the decision and its outcomes.

Nursing ethics can be said to incorporate both a set of moral principles and your personal beliefs. An understanding of both will help you to reach informed decisions in healthcare and can resolve conflicts, by allowing you to attempt to understand others' perspectives when working in a multidisciplinary team (MDT).

Ethics can be defined as a philosophical area that deals with the ethical or moral dimension of people, their actions and interactions, and the consequences of those actions and interactions.

When we think about morals and morality we tend to focus on the following points:

- judgements about right and wrong;
- respect for others;
- duty to do right for its own sake.

All of these aspects are important in the provision of healthcare and we should remember them in our normal practice. In their book of 1979 (there have been several editions since) Beauchamp and Childress first proposed the use of ethical principles in biomedical science and healthcare. They suggest that: 'A well-developed ethical theory provides a framework within which agents can reflect on the acceptability of actions and can evaluate moral judgements and moral character' (Beauchamp and Childress 1979: p. 44).

Responsible care involves the use of your own moral principles, values and beliefs taking into account the four principles outlined by Beauchamp and Childress in 1979 giving us:

- **Autonomy**: whereby a person's intrinsic value as an individual is respected, and their beliefs and basic right to self-determination is acknowledged and facilitated.
- **Beneficence**: all healthcare workers are obliged to do what is in the patient's best interests.
- **Non-maleficence**: whereby intentional or foreseeable harming of a patient is to be avoided.
- **Justice**: all patients have a right to be treated fairly and equitably regardless of social or physical position.

But in addition we should also consider in light of the 2015 NMC Code and our duty of candour:

- **Veracity**: telling the truth at all times.

Ethical behaviour and application of healthcare ethics is a complex area; however, the simple principles outlined above are easy to grasp. Our culture has firmly embraced these ethical principles in its law and in the standards our professional and regulatory body sets out for us. Self-awareness is very important and reflection in practice can help with this.

The role of the nurse

The role of the nurse from a legal, ethical and professional stance is a very important role indeed. The practising healthcare professional should be aware of the law and standards governing their practice and adhere to this law and the standards at all times. In mental health, as in other areas of healthcare provision, the nurse very often acts in an advocatory role for their patients and can be a conduit of communication for them. The relationship between the nurse and their patient is a professional one and therefore they have a duty of care to do the best for them at all times. The nurse may be asked to participate in care that needs to be given under the Mental Health Act as outlined above. They should be aware of the areas of the Act and their process of participation and involvement.

Professional guidelines and standards for practice

As we have already mentioned nurses are bound by the NMC Code of Conduct for nurses and midwives (2015) and the standards for clinical practice set out by the professional and regulatory body as well as adhering to the standards of law. These standards are expected by patients from all healthcare professionals and we as nurses represent our profession when we act in a caring role. The NMC Code is a set of values and principles to be adhered to and they can be interpreted and applied in all practice settings. As a nurse we commit to upholding these at all times and this commitment is a fundamental part of our professional persona. Nurses who act outside of the remit of, or fail to uphold, the principles of the Code are liable to action from the NMC in respect to any breach. This can result in punitive measures including conditions of practice, suspension of registration and in extreme cases removal from the register (being 'struck off'). This is why the code is so important for all nurses who care about good nursing practice.

Key learning points

Legal aspects

▸ There are many areas of law, such as The Mental Health Act and The Mental Capacity Act, relating to care of the patient with a mental health disorder and the nurse should be familiar with these and how they apply them to their area of practice.
▸ Accountability and responsibility is an important aspect of professional practice from a legal and professional perspective.
▸ Ethical behaviour is expected as part of nursing practice and is related to the nurse's responsibilities for practicing legally in healthcare.

Professional aspects

▸ The nurse has a professional responsibility to carry out their normal practice in a competent and compassionate manner.
▸ The NMC Code of Conduct should be familiar to all nurses and they should practise within its standards.

Multiple choice questions

Try answering these multiple choice questions to test what you have learned from reading this chapter. You can check your answers on page 149.

1 **What is the number of the NICE clinical guideline that contains information about the Mental Health Act?**

    a) CG76
    b) CG56

c) CG90

d) CG136

2 What year was the latest amendment to the Mental Health Act made?

a) 1959

b) 1983

c) 1995

d) 2007

3 How may consent to treatment be given?

a) Written

b) Verbal

c) Implied

d) All of the above

4 The person assessing mental capacity to consent to treatment should be

a) A healthcare professional involved in the patient's treatment

b) A judge or magistrate

c) An independent medical expert

d) The patients relative or carer

5 The 'nurse's holding power' section of the Mental Health Act allows a nurse to detain a patient for up to

a) 1 hour

b) 3 hours

c) 6 hours

d) 24 hours

6 What section of the Mental Health Act is concerned with doctor's holding power?

a) Section 3

b) Section 2

c) Section 5(2)

d) Section 5(4)

7 What is the length of time allowed for compulsory detention under section 3 of the Mental Health Act?

a) 6 hours

b) 72 hours

c) 6 months

d) Indefinite

8 Mental Health Tribunals have the power to decide

a) If a patient falls subject to the Mental Health Act
b) If a patient can continue to be detained
c) If a patient has capacity to consent
d) If a patient can have treatment

9 Which of these outline the nurse's accountability and responsibility in clinical practice?

a) The NMC Code of Conduct
b) The Mental Health Act
c) The Mental Capacity Act
d) All of the above

10 What may be the ultimate outcome for a nurse found to be in serious breach of the NMC Code of Conduct?

a) A fine
b) Loss of her job
c) Being 'struck off' the register
d) Prison

Case study

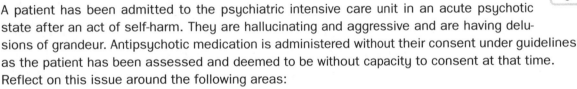

A patient has been admitted to the psychiatric intensive care unit in an acute psychotic state after an act of self-harm. They are hallucinating and aggressive and are having delusions of grandeur. Antipsychotic medication is administered without their consent under guidelines as the patient has been assessed and deemed to be without capacity to consent at that time. Reflect on this issue around the following areas:

- capacity;
- consent;
- ethics;
- professional responsibilities;
- the law.

Recommended further reading

Beauchamp, T. and Childress, L. (1979) *Principles of Biomedical Ethics*. Oxford: Oxford University Press.

Jameton, A. (1984) *Nursing Practice – The Ethical Issues*. Michigan: Prentice Hall.

MIND. *Mental Health Act 1983*. London: Mind. Available at: https://www.mind.org.uk/information-support/legal-rights/mental-health-act.aspx#.Vks2v7dyaic (accessed 19 February 2016).

National Institute for Health and Care Excellence (2012) *CG 136 Service User Experience in Adult Mental Health Services*. Available at: http://www.nccmh.org.uk/downloads/Patient%20experience/Service%20user%20experience%20full%20guidance%20published.pdf (accessed 19 February 2016).

Nursing and Midwifery Council (2015) *The Code for Nurses and Midwives*. London: NMC. Available at: http://www.nmc.org.uk/globalassets/sitedocuments/nmc-publications/revised-new-nmc-code.pdf (accessed 19 February 2016).

The Crown Office. *Mental Health Act 1983*. Available at: http://www.legislation.gov.uk/ukpga/1983/20/contents (accessed 19 February 2016).

The Crown Office. *Mental Health Act 2007*. Available at: http://www.legislation.gov.uk/ukpga/2007/12/contents (accessed 19 February 2016).

The Crown Office. *Mental Capacity Act 2005*. Available at: http://www.legislation.gov.uk/ukpga/2005/9/contents (accessed 19 February 2016).

Medicines management

3

Learning objectives

After reading this chapter you will have gained knowledge around:

- The clinical and practical relevance of medicines management.
- The role of the nurse and the MDT in medicines management.
- The frameworks that allow for non-medical prescribing.
- The factors to consider in drug administration.
- The principles of safe drug calculation.

Introduction

The concept of medicines management is not new. Helping people to take their medicines, both prescribed and over the counter, in the most appropriate way is something that nurses have been doing for many years. In 2004 the Medicines and Healthcare Products Regulatory Agency (MHRA) defined medicines management as: 'The clinical, cost-effective and safe use of medicines to ensure patients get the maximum benefit from the medicines they need, while at the same time minimizing potential harm' (MHRA 2004, as cited in NMC 2008a: p. 4).

And this is substantiated by the NMC's publication of 2008 *Standards for Medicines Management* that outlines the roles and responsibilities of the nurse and relates this to the 'duty of care' owed in caring for patients. The standards also give guidance and information on the key areas addressed by each of the 26 standards. It states:

> The administration of medicines is an important aspect of the professional practice of persons whose names are on the Council's register. It is not solely a mechanistic task to be performed in strict compliance with the written prescription of a medical practitioner (can now also be an independent and supplementary prescriber). It requires thought and the exercise of professional judgement...

> (NMC 2008a: p. 3)

The role of the nurse

The role of the nurse in medicines management is not to be underestimated. Nurses are involved in frontline patient care and spend more time with the patient than many other healthcare professionals. They are also very often responsible for drug administration and involved in patient education around the medicines prescribed. This makes them ideally placed to carry out medicines management. This can occur in a hospital or a community-based setting and the nurse should be aware at every patient or client contact that they have an oppor-

tunity to discuss medicines with them. This can be through simple enquiry or by discussion with relatives and carers involved in medicines administration. The nurse should check that the patient is still taking their medicines, that they are following the prescribed regimen and that they are having an effect from the drug without adverse or troublesome side-effects. It is important to think about how the patient or client accesses their medication and their ability to take it as well.

Clinical relevance

Why does medicines management matter? This is a question student nurses often ask but even the qualified nurse will wonder at times why they should put such an emphasis on medicines management. The complex and multifaceted area of medicines management requires all health professionals involved in a patient's prescribed medication to reach a shared understanding of medication *need* and medication *use* in conjunction with the patient. This can improve patient adherence to medication regimes and improve clinical outcomes. In November 2013 the Kings Fund Published a report on *Polypharmacy & Medicines Optimisation* (Duerden et al. 2013) and among its key findings was that many people often do not take medicines as they are intended and in fact evidence shows that many dispensed medicines are unused or wasted. The report also suggests that patients may struggle with complex drug regimens and that their perspective in medicines and medicine taking was a vital part of medicines management.

Role of the multidisciplinary team

We have already identified the role of the nurse in medicines management but it is important to remember that few healthcare professionals function alone. Many of us work as part of a MDT and we all play a role within that team in caring for the patients and clients we are responsible for. In establishing which role we play within the team we can then see how the nurse can function as an effective member of that team for the good of patient care. This role will depend on the area you work in *and* the level you are practising at. The role of a student nurse within the team is very different from that of an advanced nurse practitioner and therefore responsibilities will vary.

Reflective exercise

Think about your current role and identify it within the MDT you work with. Consider how the performance of your role and responsibilities impacts on other members of the team. Reflect on areas such as team meetings, role boundaries and patient involvement. Apply this to the area of medicines management.

Changing role in practice

The role we play in medicines management will change as our career evolves. But from our time as a student nurse up to that of staff nurse, ward manager, advanced practitioner or nursing lecturer, we still have a part to play in this important area of client and patient care. This is not to say that our role is any less or any more important as our career develops, often just 'different'. The reflective exercise above should have clarified your current role in your mind and helped you to analyse the roles of other members of the team. Understanding that your role will change as your career progresses is important in all aspects of care but more so in medicines management. It is not expected that a student nurse would act autonomously in this role but it is essential they are involved and can gain good understanding and insight into the importance of it from mentors and senior colleagues. Often the nurse acts as an advocate or 'patient voice' in this area creating a bridge of communication between the patient and prescriber. This role is common to all members of the team as even the perceived 'least' responsible in this area can highlight issues that need to be addressed. The knowledge that bringing a medicines issue to the prescriber's attention is as important as changing a medication is something that should be instilled at the earliest point of nurse

training and should stay with us throughout our working lives.

Non-medical prescribing

Non-medical prescribing is now well established within the UK. However, until the Cumberledge Report, *Neighbourhood Nursing: A Focus for Care* (Department of Health and Social Security 1986) suggested that prescribing rights be extended, it did not exist, and indeed the healthcare system has gone through many changes to bring us to the present day situation. Today suitably qualified nurses, pharmacists and certain other allied health professionals can prescribe independently from the whole *British National Formulary* (BNF), within their area of clinical competence, including unlicensed medicine and some controlled drugs. This role does not extend to all nurses, pharmacists and allied health professionals and indeed the professional wishing to become a non-medical prescriber must meet rigorous entry criteria to the training course required by the professional and regulatory bodies, for them to become eligible to be recorded as a non-medical prescriber.

The nurse in their role as drug administrator will be liaising with prescribers from all the non-medical prescribing professions as well as doctors and needs to be familiar with the range and type of prescribing that each healthcare professional can carry out. This involves good communication with prescribers in the nurse's clinical area and clear delineation of prescriber roles and responsibilities.

The team approach

Knowing that we all have a role within the MDT is the first step in ensuring a team approach to medicines management. A well-functioning and cohesive team approach to patient-centred care is essential in optimizing medicine-taking behaviour in our patients and involving all appropriate parties in decisions about medicines, their use and in prescribing, dispensing and administration duties. Knowing that you are 'not on your own' but have the support and supervision of other team members can ensure that knowledge and learning are well managed and patient safety is prioritized. This team approach also has a bearing on the patient's ability to adhere to medication regimes and therefore improve patient outcomes. Feeling that there are many people involved in the decisions about their medicines can improve patient confidence in the appropriateness of treatment. Knowing a doctor or other qualified prescriber has taken account of pharmacist knowledge and input gives the patient faith that the medication is truly appropriate and that any interactions or cautions have been duly considered. Knowing that the nurse who looks after them daily and knows their routine and lifestyle also has involvement helps them trust the regime designed for them. Good communication is key to this happening.

Factors in administration

The NMC clearly states that as a registered nurse you are accountable for your actions and omissions (NMC 2008b). This includes administration of medicines and reminds nurses that they must think through issues *and* that the nurse must apply their professional expertise and judgment in the best interests of the patient. It is also for nurses to remember that even if there is joint responsibility for drug administration they remain accountable for their own actions. One of the fundamentals of safe drug administration is knowledge around the medicine to be given. This includes:

■ the therapeutic indication;
■ the normal dose range;

■ the possible side effects;
■ the presence of any cautions or contraindications;
■ the potential for drug interaction;
■ the allergy status of the patient.

It is also important that local policies and procedures are adhered to when medication is being administered. This includes the 'Five Rights' shown in Figure 3.1.

The right patient

It is vital to ensure you have the correct patient before administration of any medication. This involves confirming identity with the patient verbally where they have capacity to do so and checking details with the patient identification bracelet if present. These details should be compared with the medication prescription chart to verify the *right patient* receives the medication.

The right medication

Most medications have at least two names, the generic name (and where no issues exist this is how it should be prescribed) and the brand name(s). Some drug packaging will carry both names and it is the responsibility of the administrator to verify that the *right medication* is given. It is important that the nurse knows what the drug is given to treat and this can be checked in the BNF.

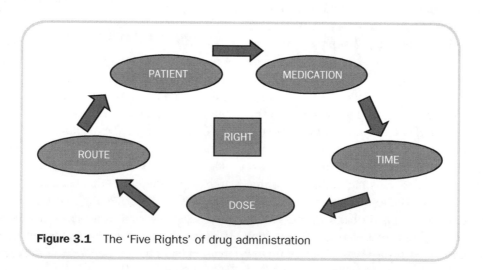

Figure 3.1 The 'Five Rights' of drug administration

The right time

Drugs are often prescribed at set times in hospital settings and drug rounds are done to coincide with these timings. But for medication that is taken as required, one-off doses or in the community dosing schedules should be adhered to. If a drug is required three times per day then these three doses should be evenly spaced throughout the day time (or night if specified by the prescriber) and maximum daily doses should never be exceeded. This ensures the medicines are given at the *right time*.

The right dose

This is where skill in drug calculation often comes into play. The drug may be written up as a set dose but the nurse may have different strength tablets to supply and calculation is then required of how many tablets are needed. The drug may be prescribed as a certain amount of milligrams per kilogram and the nurse must work out the dose based on the patient's weight. This is to ensure that the *right dose* is administered. This is covered in more detail in the drug calculation section to follow.

The right route

It is vital that the prescriber states on the prescription the *right route* for drug administration to allow the nurse to give the drug the way it was intended. Oral medications are the most common and error with route in these cases is rare. But drugs to be given by injection must have the injection route stated so the administrator knows whether this injection is intravenous (IV), intramuscular (IM) or subcutaneous (SC). Clear direction for route should be seen.

Introduction to drug calculation

It is a widely accepted fact that nurses need to have the skill to perform safe and accurate drug calculations in their everyday practice. This skill is required mainly in their role of safe drug administration. It is therefore vital that nurses begin to engage with arithmetic and mathematics early in their education and carry this skill through into all areas of their career. This introduction to safe drug calculation will start you on this journey and give you the basic tools to help you to engage with other purpose-designed texts to develop and maintain your ability in this area.

Standard international unit conversion

Before performing many drug calculations you must be able to convert the numbers you use in the calculation so that they all appear in the same standard international (SI) units. You need to be familiar with these units; they are the most common that will be encountered in performing drug calculations as they will be written on the prescription charts that you use. In Box 3.1 you will see the commonest SI units involved in medicines administration, their approved abbreviation (or symbol) and their equivalent in the next unit of size. You should be able to convert easily and confidently between these units of mass before attempting to move on to the area of drug calculation formula that follows in this section – so spend some time doing the practice conversions that are here for you.

■ To convert from a smaller unit to the next higher unit *divide* by 1000
■ To convert from a larger unit to a smaller unit *multiply* by 1000

This process is best illustrated by the use of examples.

If we want to convert from a smaller unit (in this case a milligram) to a larger unit (for example a gram) you need to *divide* by 1000, so:

$$10,000\text{mg} \div 1000 = 10\text{g}$$

To convert from a larger unit (in the example shown here a gram) to a smaller unit (a milligram) you should *multiply* by 1000, so:

$$10\text{g} \times 1000 = 10,000\text{mg}$$

There are some conversion practice questions at the end of this chapter to help you master this skill. Use these before you move onto the next section if you are unsure.

The basic formula method for drug calculation

There are many ways in arithmetical text that can be used to perform drug calculations, but the

Box 3.1 Standard International (SI) units

Unit	Symbol	Equivalent	Symbol
1 kilogram	kg	1000 grams	g
1 gram	g	1000 milligrams	mg
1 milligram	mg	1000 micrograms	mcg or μg*
1 microgram	mcg	1000 nanograms	ng

*These symbols should not be used in good practice – micrograms should always be written in full.

simplest and most widely used method is the basic formula method which is shown here:

$$\frac{D \times Q}{H} = X$$

Where:

- D = desired dose
- H = strength available
- Q = quantity or unit of measure (for tablets Q = 1; for liquids Q can vary)
- X = dose to be determined/amount to be given

But many nurses know this formula in another guise:

$$\frac{WYW}{WYG} \times WII = X$$

Where:

- WYW = what you want = desired dose
- WYG = what you've got = strength available
- WII = what it is in = quantity or unit of measure (for tablets this = 1; for liquids it can vary)
- X = dose to be determined/amount to be given

Whichever way you remember the equation above the steps for using the basic formula method are as follows:

- first, memorize the formula;
- remember to convert all the numbers involved to the same SI unit;
- place all of the numbers into the correct place within the basic formula;
- calculate your answer;
- label all your answers (for example tablets, capsules, ml).

Here are two examples; work through them and check your answers at each stage with the ones given.

1. Your patient needs Drug A at a dose of 1g to be given as an oral tablet.

   You have 250 milligram tablets.

   How many tablets should you give?

   $$1g \times 1000 = 1000mg$$

   $$1000/250 \times 1 = 4 \text{ tablets}$$

2. Your patient requires 600mg of Drug B, which comes as a liquid to be given orally.

   You have a 150mg/2ml strength of solution.

   What volume of drug should be given?

   $$600/150 \times 2 = 8ml$$

   Here are some more examples of how to do calculations with specific criteria.

Drug calculations involving solid doses of medication

Your patient requires 1.6g of a drug every six hours (four times per day). You have 400mg tablets and need to calculate the number of tablets per dose, per day and for a seven-day supply.

- How many tablets per dose?

First we convert the units:

$$1.6g \times 1000 = 1600mg$$

$1600\,(D)\,/400\,(H) \times 1\,(Q) = 4$ tablets per dose (X)

■ How many tablets per day?

Now we know how many per dose we can move on:

4 tablets × 4 (times per day) = 16 tablets per day

■ How many tablets for a seven-day supply?

Now we know how many per day we can move on:

16 tablets × 7 (days) = 112 tablets for a seven-day supply

Drug calculations involving liquid doses of medication

Your patient requires 750mg of a drug three times per day. You have 150mg in 5ml strength liquid and you need to calculate how much per dose, per day and for a five-day supply.

■ How many ml per dose?

There is no SI unit conversion needed so we use the formula now. But note Q in this equation = 5

$750(D)/150(H) \times 5(Q) = 25$ml per dose

■ How many ml per day?

We know how many ml for one dose so we can move on:

25ml × 3 (times per day) = 75ml per day

■ How many ml for a five-day supply?

We know how many ml for one day so we can move on:

75ml × 5 (days) = 375ml for a five-day supply

Drug calculations involving weight

Your patient requires a drug at a dose of 60mg per kg per day. They weigh 12kg and you have 120mg/5ml liquid. This needs to be given four times per day. You need to calculate how much per day based on weight and then how much per dose.

■ How much per day based on weight?

$60(mg) \times 12(kg) \times 1\,(day) = 720$mg per day

■ How much per dose?

$720(mg)\,/4$ (times per day) = 180mg per dose

Drug calculations involving time

Your patient requires a drug at a dose of 2g as a once only dose. You have 400mg/2ml strength liquid for IV injection. The dose needs to be given at a rate of 1ml every 30 seconds.

■ How many ml for the dose?

$$2g \times 1000 = 2000mg$$

$$2000(D)/400(H) \times 2\,(Q) = 10\text{ml for the dose}$$

■ How long to give the dose?

1ml every 30 seconds = 2ml every minute

10ml/2ml = 5 minutes

This should now give you the necessary skills to be able to attempt the practice questions at the end of this and each relevant chapter.

In this chapter we have looked at the concept of medicines management and your role as the nurse within a MDT in this important area of healthcare practice. Look over the key learning points and try the drug calculations and multiple choice questions to test your learning. Then consider the points in the case study to apply your learning to practice.

Key learning points

Medicines management

▶ The nurse plays a vital role in medicines management.
▶ The role of the nurse is outlined in the NMC *Standards for Medicines Management*. ⟶

←
▶ The nurse functions in this role as part of a MDT.
▶ Improving adherence and patient outcomes is central in medicines management.

Drug calculations

▶ The ability to perform safe and accurate drug calculations is central to a nurse's role.
▶ Application of numerical ability to practical drug administration settings is vital.

Drug calculations

1 How many milligrams are there in 4g?

2 How many micrograms are there in 2.75mg?

3 How many nanograms are there in 0.3 micrograms?

4 How many grams are there in 475mg?

5 How many milligrams are there in 800 micrograms?

6 Your patient is prescribed 1g of drug A. You have 500mg tablets.

How many tablets for one dose?

7 Your patient is prescribed 2.4g of drug B. You have 600mg tablets.

How many tablets for one dose?

8 Your patient is prescribed 360mg of drug C. You have 120mg/5ml strength liquid.

How many ml for one dose?

9 Your patient is prescribed 250 micrograms of drug D. You have 62.5 micrograms/2ml strength liquid.

How many ml for one dose?

10 Your patient is prescribed 0.1g of drug E. You have 50mg/2ml strength solution for injection.

How many ml for one dose?

Multiple choice questions
Try answering these multiple choice questions to test what you have learned from reading this chapter. You can check your answers on page 150.

1 The NMC relates the responsibility of the nurse in medicines management to their

   a) Duty of Honesty
   b) Duty of Care

←

c) Duty of Competence
d) Duty of Ability

2 What does the Kings Fund report of 2013 suggest?

a) Patients don't like medicines
b) Patients struggle to understand instructions
c) Patients struggle with complex medicines regimes
d) Prescribers don't make doses clear

3 What is key to an effective team approach to medicines management?

a) Good knowledge
b) Good meetings
c) Good work environment
d) Good communication

4 What are the main factors in drug administration?

a) The five rights
b) The four rights
c) The avoidance of harm principle
d) The code of conduct

5 In medicines management, what are the units of measurement, including the units of mass, known as

a) SI units
b) IS units
c) Kg
d) Milligrams

6 What is the safest way to calculate drug doses?

a) In your head
b) Using the basic formula method
c) Asking a pharmacist to do it
d) From memory

7 What can a nurse use to check a medication is being given to the correct patient?

a) Patient name band
b) Patient verbally confirming details
c) Drug prescription chart
d) All of the above

8 How should a nurse check what a drug is used to treat?

a) The patient drug prescription chart

→

b) In the BNF

c) Ask the patient

d) Guess

9 How should micrograms be written on a prescription chart?

a) It does not need to be written

b) As mg

c) As μg

d) As micrograms

10 What is the SI unit for nanograms?

a) ng

b) NG

c) Nanog

d) Nang

Case study

You are a student nurse doing a drug round with your mentor in a busy hospital ward. You come to a patient and the drug they are prescribed is not one you have ever heard of. Your mentor asks you how you should safely proceed to administer the patient's medication. What factors would you consider before giving the patient their medication?

Recommended website

British National Formulary (BNF) www.bnf.org

Recommended further reading

Department of Health and Social Security (1986), *Neighbourhood Nursing: A Focus for Care. The Cumberledge Report*. London: Department of Health and Social Security.

Duerden, M., Avery, T. & Payne, R. (2013) *Polypharmacy and Medicines Optimisation* published by the Kings Fund: London.

Lapham, R. & Agr, H. (2009) *Drug Calculations for Nurses, 3rd edn*. London: Arnold.

Nursing & Midwifery Council (NMC) (2008a) *Standards for Medicines Management*. London: NMC.

Nursing & Midwifery Council (NMC) (2008b) *The Code: Standards of Conduct, Performance and Ethics for Nurses and Midwives*. London: NMC.

Rogers, K. & Scott, W (2011) *Nurses! Test Yourself in Essential Calculation Skills*. Maidenhead: Open University Press.

Shihab, P. (2014) *Numeracy in Nursing & Healthcare – Calculations and Practice, 2nd edn*. London: Routledge.

Medicines adherence and the therapeutic alliance

4

Learning objectives

After reading this chapter you will have gained knowledge around:

- The principles of adherence, compliance and concordance.
- The role of the nurse in medicine-taking behaviour.
- The importance of the patient at the centre of medicines management.
- The strategies that can be used to optimize medicine taking and adherence.
- The importance of carer and client involvement.

Introduction

The guidance on medicines adherence produced in NICE's CG76 defines medicines adherence as enabling patients to make informed choices by involving and supporting them in decisions about prescribed medicines (NICE 2009). It goes on to discuss what is adherence and how can it be achieved. Put simply, 'Adherence to medicines is defined as the extent to which the patient's behaviour matches the agreed recommendations' (NICE 2009: p. 1).

When we look at the traditional role of the doctor as a prescriber, they are often viewed as paternalistic and authoritative in their relationship with patients taking their medicines. This is no longer a valid or widely accepted model for medicines management. We actively encourage our patients to participate, where possible and desired by them, in the decision making around medication prescription and choice. Where patients feel actively involved in medication initiation and continuation they are more likely to adhere to the regime agreed with the consequence of improved outcomes.

In the arena of medicine-taking behaviour you will be familiar with the word adherence as it is a commonly used term regarding the extent to which patients take their medicines and is something we as healthcare professionals can measure. You may also come across other terms that you should be familiar with, and two terms will be explained below.

Compliance

The word 'comply', as understood by many people, means 'doing as instructed' or 'doing what you are told'. This is not incorrect and compliance is a term often used to mean this; however, we must be careful to always do so in a positive manner. The word itself can make us think of a passivity and obedience. Patients and clients do not like to feel they are being described as non-compliant as this has negative behaviour connotations. This can lead to feelings of unease and a strain within the therapeutic alliance with their healthcare professional. It does describe the *degree* to which

a patient *correctly* follows medical advice, which is why it is still used but it has largely been superseded by the use of the term 'adherence'. Non-compliance can take two forms, direct and indirect.

In direct non-compliance the patient wilfully chooses not to follow the medical advice given around their medicines and how they should be taken. It is more common in patients who do not take medicines prescribed for them at all but also accounts for some patients who do not take them as they were intended to be administered (over- and under-medication, poor timings, missed doses).

In indirect non-compliance, there is often no wilful choice to deviate from the prescriber's instructions but the medicine-taking behaviour does not follow the advice or regime set. This can be through poor patient knowledge of the medicines and their regime, lack of understanding about the doses or scheduling or poor communication between prescriber and patient. The outcome is usually an incorrect regime of administration that may lead to poorer outcomes.

Reflective exercise

Think about patients or clients you have worked with that have been described as 'non-compliant' and why this may be the case.

Concordance

Concordance relates to the involvement of the patient in the decision-making process, where possible, as an equal partner, whose views, beliefs and input have as much influence on the medication prescribed and plan of treatment as that of the healthcare professional. It involves negotiation between the parties involved to reach an *agreed* outcome that respects both the clinical need and the patient's wishes.

It requires a good therapeutic alliance between the healthcare professional and the patient where effective communication is essential. Patients do, however, choose not to participate in or are unable to participate in the decision-making process for many reasons and therefore true concordance is not achievable. This is certainly the case with children, adults who lack capacity to understand or consent (those with mental capacity issues or those unconscious or anaesthetized) or patients who simply prefer their prescriber to make the decisions for them. A choice to not participate is just as much the patient's right as participation. It was thought that concordance was the optimum way of ensuring correct medication-taking behaviour but an experienced and self-aware practitioner can elicit information through the use of open and closed consultation techniques, including behavioural observation, to get a 'feel' for how the prescription of medications would impact on a patient's life and then tailor the medications regimes in a more appropriate manner. Concordance is and was an ideal; adherence is a much more realistic way of approaching medicine-taking behaviour and is now more favoured in prescribing circles.

The importance of adherence

The therapeutic alliance has been seen in the past as very much like what we have discussed above and probably takes into account aspects of concordance, compliance and adherence rather than being closely modelled on any one of the three. It does and should involve the patient to the extent they can participate and wish to be involved. Their rights to autonomy within the relationship should be maintained while seeking their views, beliefs and input at every appropriate point. It not only involves the patient and their prescriber but can incorporate anyone else involved in care around medicine. This is typically the pharmacist who is dispensing, the nurse who is administering and the carers or family members involved either in a hospital setting or at home.

If adherence is the patient taking medication as it is prescribed then the importance of this cannot be understated. With a significant medication input into the management of mental health conditions it is vital that the patients take these medications in order to improve the chance of recovery and a better quality of life. Many of these medications need to be taken as they are prescribed to maintain consistent blood levels of the drug to produce optimal therapeutic effect. Any lapse in adherence can lead to a relapse of symptoms that can prove detrimental to the patient's chances of recovery. It can also lead to hospital admission, risk of suicide or self-harm and jeopardize treatment plans.

Many people equate non-adherence with patients not taking their medication at all, but this is too simplistic. Patients may change when they take their medicines, how they take them or may over-dose themselves (not necessarily intentionally) by playing around with the regime set by the prescriber.

Medicines that are prescribed for the patient but are subsequently not taken by them represents a significant economic burden to the NHS, both in the cost of the drugs themselves and the perceived waste of medical time (Cushing and Metcalfe 2007).

Adherence is a complex mix of many different factors and cannot be viewed as a singular entity. Many other factors may occur that are very specific to that patient at that time and need to be included in the decision-making process. Some of the things we need to consider can be seen in Box 4.1. The list is by no means exhaustive but is a good place for you to start.

> **Box 4.1 Factors that influence adherence**
>
> - Social factors
> - Access to medicines – prescriptions and dispensing
> - Cost of prescriptions to patients
> - Patient's views, attitudes and beliefs
> - Level of understanding
> - The disease itself
> - Comorbidities and other medications
> - Previous experiences with medicines
> - Communication

Case example

If we consider a patient, Mary, with regard to the factors that may influence her adherence we would need a range of information to help us identify if any of the factors above apply.
Mary is 84 years old and currently lives alone in a sheltered housing complex. Her husband died ten years ago and her only son lives in Australia with his family. She has had a hip replacement and suffers from osteoarthritis. She is also suffering from dementia and although these are early stages in the disease she has memory problems. She needs daily medication for her dementia as well as for her pain.

Consider Mary and which factors are influential and why. Once you have come up with your answers, see the box on p. 35 of this chapter for our suggestions.

The role of the nurse

As outlined previously, the nurse is ideally placed to contribute to helping the patient to take their medication as it is prescribed.

One of the important roles of the nurse is to assess and monitor adherence. This can be done in many ways.

- Asking the patient – get them to report to you on their perception of their adherence to the medication regime.
- Ask the family – carers and family members can report on the patient's behalf.
- Count up unused medicines and relate these to the dispensing date to see if all doses have been taken.
- Patient records – these can be hospital, general practitioner (GP) or pharmacy.
- Blood or urine tests for therapeutic levels.

All these methods can help to give a good approximation of the level of adherence but unless you are actually administering the medications, a full profile of adherence is difficult to achieve.

Incorporating health beliefs and patient choice

Very many of the patients you encounter will have their own set of values and beliefs around health. This is normal and to be expected, as it is normal for their beliefs and views to be different from your own. It is, however, important that you remember that the patient should be at the centre of all considerations around their care.

Strategies to optimize adherence

There are many strategies that the nurse can employ in their quest to optimize medicines adherence. One of the strongest is a good rapport or a therapeutic alliance with the patient as we have discussed above. This is not restricted to the prescriber and patient but involves all partners in the patient's care. There are many other strategies that can be employed. See below for some examples of the most effective.

1. Simplify medicine regimes. A drug regime where the medicine is to be taken once daily is more likely to be adhered to than one where a drug should be given four times per day.

2. Only prescribe when necessary. This seems like stating the obvious but unnecessary prescriptions or over-the-counter medicines should be avoided.

3. Avoid polypharmacy. The more drugs a patient has to take the more chance there is for confusion, error or non-adherence.

4. Choose packaging and formulation carefully to consider the patient's ability to get into medicines and take them appropriately.

5. Check ease of access to prescriptions and medications and help with organizing delivery and collection where available.

6. Educate the patient on the areas of drug effects, side-effects, potential adverse effects and effects of non-adherence.

7. Provide information that can be written, verbal, recorded, in braille or large print or translated if necessary. It is important that the information is in the medium most suitable for the patient.

8. Carer and family involvement, to ensure that people in the home also know about the medicines.

9. Positivity of attitude from you can influence the patient's attitude to medicine taking.

10. Effective consultation management including environment, time spent and opportunity to ask questions.

11. Regular review and monitoring to check for effects expected and any side-effects.

12. Reflection on each consultation to ensure safe and consistent practice and to evaluate the healthcare professional–patient interaction.

Client and carer involvement

This is an area that can be overlooked in the medicines management of our patients and clients but is often very important, especially in caring for children and adolescents, elderly people and those with reduced mental capacity for any reason. Clients or patients are encouraged to be involved, as we have discussed earlier in this chapter, looking at partnership and influence in decision making, but should also be involved at review and monitoring stages and, if able, they should be encouraged to self-manage where appropriate. Carers can be paid carers in someone's home environment or, as is more often the case, family or friends who are responsible for some or all of the home care of the patient. Regardless of category, they should be consulted and involved where and when it is prudent to do so and with the consent if needed of the patient. In the area of mental healthcare, the family, relatives, friends and carers often can and will act as advocates for the patient when they are less able to be involved in their care. As long as it is appropriate for them to do so they can be invaluable aids in the decision-making process around initiation and continuation of medications. They are well-placed to give information about the patient that can assist in choosing the best and most appropriate medicines to be prescribed.

In this chapter we have looked at the therapeutic alliance and its importance in medicines management. We have also explored the concept of adherence to medicines and how important the role of the mental health nurse is in this area.

Look over the key learning points and try the drug calculations and multiple choice questions to test your learning. Then consider the points in the case study to apply your learning to practice.

Case example – suggested responses

■ Social factors – Mary lives alone but has someone popping in as she is in sheltered housing, so we would find out if she has a good social network of friends. Does she have a social worker?

■ Access to medicines, prescriptions and dispensing – Mary may have trouble getting to the chemist, and if so can her medicines be delivered?

■ Cost of prescriptions to patients – should not be an issue as she is entitled to free prescriptions due to her age.

■ Patient's views, attitudes and beliefs – Mary would need to be involved as much as possible in her medicines management so that these can be taken into account.　→

←

■ Level of understanding – she needs to be informed and educated around her medicines and her understanding checked.

■ The disease itself – the dementia and memory problems may be a significant factor to consider.

■ Comorbidities and other medications – her pain and mobility are an issue and we must look at her pain medication for interactions.

■ Previous experiences with medicines – this would need to be assessed.

■ Communication – this should be paramount to establish a rapport and for assessment.

Key learning points

Medicines adherence

▶ The nurse plays a vital role in medicines adherence due to the prominent frontline role in patient care and medicines administration.

▶ Concordance, compliance and adherence are often used to describe patient medicine-taking behaviour and you should be familiar with all three.

▶ Good communication is essential in the medicines adherence process.

▶ Many strategies can be employed to optimize adherence.

Therapeutic alliance

▶ The patient should be as involved as they want to be in managing their own care.

▶ Communication and establishment of a rapport is essential to influence medicines adherence.

▶ The therapeutic alliance may involve a range of healthcare professionals, the patient, their relatives and carers.

Drug calculations

1 Your patient is prescribed 200mg of drug A every 12 hours. You have 50mg tablets.

How many tablets for one dose?

How many tablets for one day?

2 Your patient is prescribed 600mg of drug B four times per day. You have 300mg tablets.

How many tablets for one dose?

How many tablets for one day?

3 Your patient is prescribed 3g of drug C every eight hours. You have 500mg tablets.

How many tablets for one dose?

How many tablets for one day?

←

4 Your patient is prescribed 800mg of drug D daily in four divided doses. You have 100mg tablets.

How many tablets for one dose?

How many tablets for one day?

5 Your patient is prescribed 375mg of drug E every six hours. You have 0.125g/5ml strength liquid.

How many ml for one dose?

How many ml for one day?

6 Your patient is prescribed 1.25g of drug F twice daily. You have 250mg/2ml strength liquid.

How many ml for one dose?

How many ml for one day?

7 Your patient is prescribed 500mg of drug G as a bolus dose at a rate of 1ml every ten seconds. You have 250mg/5ml solution for injection.

How many ml for the dose and how long will it take to administer?

8 Your patient is prescribed 20mg of drug H. You have 2mg/ml strength liquid.

How many ml per dose?

9 Your patient is prescribed 4.5mg of drug I. You have 1.5mg/ml solution for injection.

How many ml per dose?

10 Your patient is prescribed 80mg of drug J. You have 20mg/5ml strength liquid.

How many ml per dose?

Multiple choice questions

Try answering these multiple choice questions to test what you have learned from reading this chapter. You can check your answers on page 151.

1 What is the number of the NICE clinical guideline relating to medicines adherence?

a) CG76
b) CG56
c) CG90
d) CG101

2 What should a therapeutic alliance involve?

a) The prescriber
b) The patient
c) The pharmacist
d) All of the above

3 Non-adherence is about patients not taking their medicines at all. Is this statement true?

a) True
b) False
c) Partially true; this is one form of non-adherence
d) Only if the patient lacks capacity

4 Non-adherence can lead to

a) Return of symptoms
b) Compliance
c) Concordance
d) Better outcomes

5 The roles of the nurse in adherence involve

a) Assessment
b) Monitoring
c) Education
d) All of the above

6 What is the best form of information giving for patient medications?

a) Written leaflets
b) Audio recorded
c) The one the patient requests
d) Sending them to the pharmacist

7 Reflecting on patient consultations can

a) Make the patient adhere
b) Help you evaluate patient/professional interaction
c) Reduce polypharmacy
d) Avoid the need for review

8 Which of the following relates to concordance?

a) Agreement of patient and prescriber
b) Prescriber sets agenda and terms
c) Patient sets agenda and terms
d) The need for a contract

9 Strategies to improve adherence include

a) Simpler regimes
b) Clear instructions

c) Regular review

d) All of the above

10 In direct non-compliance, the patient

a) Chooses not to take medicines as prescribed

b) Makes an error in dosing

c) Forgets to collect a prescription

d) Is unable to make a decision due to reduced capacity

Case study

You are a nurse representing the patient you have been caring for and are in discussion with a junior doctor around the medication they wish to commence despite this being against the wishes of the patient. The patient believes in herbal remedies and complementary medicine and has stopped taking their current antipsychotic drugs. They have read that prescribed drugs do not work and are adamant that a herbal supplement will suffice.

Reflect on how the patient's need for medication and their health beliefs may be reconciled for the best chance of adherence.

Recommended website

Patient Connect: http://www.patientconnect.eu/?gclid=COXnxt3PtsICFTLJtAodiAcAVA
Note: This is a useful information site around compliance.

Recommended further reading

Cushing, A. and Metcalfe, R. (2007) Optimising medicines management – from compliance to concordance. Therapeutics and clinical risk management. *Therapeutics and Clinical Risk Management* 3(6): 1047–1058.

National Institute for Health and Care Excellence (NICE) (2009) *Medicines Adherence. CG76*. London: NICE. Available at: http://www.nice.org.uk/guidance/cg76 (accessed 21 February 2016).

Anatomy and physiology of the brain

5

Chapter contents

Learning objectives

After reading this chapter you will have gained knowledge around:

- The structure and function of the normal human brain.
- The principles of neurotransmission and the function of the synapse.
- The role and function of brain monoamines.
- The impact of altered physiology.

Introduction

It is important to have a full understanding of the pathophysiology involved in mental health disorders and subsequent pharmacological interventions. In order to develop this knowledge you should first have a good grounding in the basic anatomy and physiology of the brain. The brain is the site of the altered physiology and function that underlies many of the common mental health disorders and many conditions are linked to specific anomalies.

This chapter will not go into in-depth neuroanatomical detail but will give you a sufficient overview of structure and function to aid your learning and understanding. The brain is probably the most complex organ in the human body with many areas, tissues, cells and chemicals involved in its functionality. For many years very little was known about the brain as anatomy was derived from post-mortem dissections, but with increasing levels of technology and scanning available today, more is known about the discrete areas of the brain and their functional aspects. We will look at the different brain regions and cells and discuss neurotransmission and the monoamines and chemicals involved.

Structure of the brain

The organ known as the brain is structured into regions (Figure 5.1). Each region can be seen as distinct when we look at diagrammatic representations but there is a complex system of connections between the regions to make up the brain itself. We will look at each main brain region in turn.

Cerebral cortex (cerebrum)

This is the largest part of the brain and it is separated anatomically and functionally into four lobes spanning two hemispheres (left and right). The lobes are:

- frontal;
- parietal;
- occipital;
- temporal.

It is a 'wrinkled' structure in appearance and due to these folds has a large surface area despite the size of the brain itself being relatively small and restricted by the skull. It is also defined into two areas by colour, these being the grey and the white matter. The grey matter is the outer layer, that which is visible on the surface of the brain

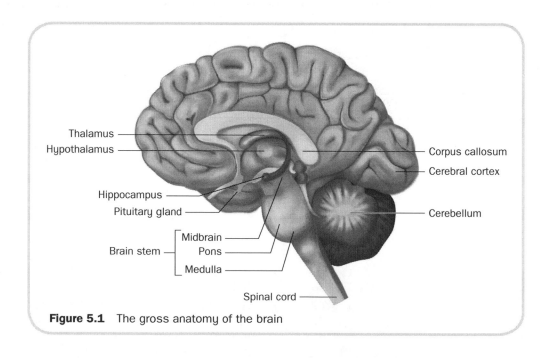

Figure 5.1 The gross anatomy of the brain

and this is made up of nerve cell bodies and dendrites (see more on neuron structure below). The white matter is found in the deeper tissue of the brain and is made up mostly of the axonal portions of the nerve cells.

Cerebellum

The cerebellum (or little brain) is located at the lower rear of the cortex. It is anatomically a separate looking structure although very much connected to the rest of the brain. It is not wrinkled like the cortex, but more 'lined' in appearance, which is due to the tissue being arranged in a concertina-like fashion. It is made up of more than one type of nerve cell and is responsible for many different functions largely around motor function and control.

Brain stem

The brain stem is made up of three distinct parts:

- midbrain;
- pons;
- medulla oblongata.

These parts are all connected in a vertical manner with the midbrain at the top, the pons in the middle, and the medulla oblongata at the bottom which is connected to the spinal cord at the point it exits the skull. The brain stem acts to coordinate many of the higher functions of the brain and the body and is a very important structure. Its position at the base of the brain does mean it is vulnerable to compression in the event of brain injury and swelling.

Corpus callosum

The corpus callosum is essentially a thick 'bundle' of connecting nerve tissue that unites the two hemispheres of the brain. It is responsible for the relaying of information and impulses between the left and right sides.

Limbic system and the diencephalon

The limbic system and diencephalon are linked areas of the brain that consist mainly of the amygdala, thalamus, hypothalamus, hippocampus and other smaller structures. There are numerous and complex connections and interconnections between these structures and there is some debate as to whether they are in fact interrelated systems or discrete structures with good communication pathways. As you can see from Figure 5.1 they are located in close proximity to one another underneath the cerebral cortex and above the cerebellum and brain stem. They are located in the midline between the two hemispheres and beneath the corpus callosum.

Function of the brain

Each area of the brain is responsible for coordination of many functions. These can be seen in summary in Table 5.1.

Functions of the brain regions

Each lobe of the brain is responsible for different functions. Disorders of, or trauma to, the brain in specific regions can lead to specific deficits.

Cerebral cortex

This area of the brain is responsible for a great variety of functions as you can see from Table 5.1. These functions are motor, sensory and cognitive in nature. Important higher functions such as language, thought, initiation of movement and visual and auditory processing are controlled here. Many of these functions can be found to span both of the hemispheres of the brain but some functions are specific to either the left or right side; for example Broca's area, which is responsible for language processing, is found in the dominant hemisphere of the brain (for most people this is the left side).

Cerebellum

The cerebellum is mainly responsible for control of much of our motor functions. It is also involved in controlling the body's movement in the specific areas of coordination and timing of movement. It is known to have functions in areas where precision and accuracy of movement are necessary such as maintaining balance and posture.

Table 5.1   Summary of the main functions of the regions of the brain

Brain region	Summary of main functions
Cortex	**Frontal Lobe** – reasoning, planning, parts of speech, movement, emotional processing and problem-solving **Parietal lobe** – movement, orientation, recognition, processing of a variety of received stimuli **Occipital lobe** – processing of visual stimuli **Temporal lobe** – processing of auditory stimuli, memory, speech processing
Cerebellum	Movement and posture, balance
Brain stem	**Midbrain** – vision, hearing, movement **Pons** – motor and sensory functions **Medulla oblongata** – breathing and heart rate
Corpus callosum	Communicates between two hemispheres of brain
Limbic system and diencephalon	**Amygdala** – memory, emotion and fear **Hippocampus** – learning and memory **Thalamus** – motor and sensory functions **Hypothalamus** – motivation, hunger, thirst, emotion

Midbrain

The midbrain, as part of the brain stem, has been associated with some functions related to movement, such as those of the eye, but it is believed that it is more involved in the relaying of information required to process visual and auditory stimuli. This allows the brain to interpret stimuli from the eyes and ears and use this to coordinate other actions.

Pons

The pons, as part of the brain stem, has motor and sensory functions. It also acts as a relay station for signals that are being transmitted from structures above and below. These signals are primarily concerned with sleep, respiration (the pons houses the pneumotaxic centre that regulates this) and some voluntary movement.

Medulla oblongata

The medulla oblongata is the final section of the brain stem and is connected to the spinal cord at the point it exits the skull. It is involved in involuntary movement control (for example sneezing) and some reflex actions but also control of autonomic functions essential for life such as breathing, heartbeat and the maintenance of blood pressure.

Amygdala

The amygdala is part of the limbic system and is involved in emotional responses, often related to external stimuli. It plays a part in fear and phobia but also is involved in pleasure responses. Abnormal amygdala function has been linked to anxiety disorders and depression. There have also been links to memory and especially around the forming of new memories.

Hippocampus

This area of the brain is linked with memory and emotion, much like the amygdala is. It also forms part of the limbic system and is involved in short-term and long-term memory processing as well as playing a part in spatial awareness and orientation. The hippocampus allows us to form memories based on things we have experienced or encountered and is involved in the retention of these memories.

Thalamus

The thalamus is near the centre of the brain and has many functions. It is involved in sensory perception and processing as well as relaying information about these to other areas of the brain. It therefore plays a part in the senses of sight, sound and touch and some of our voluntary responses to these senses.

Hypothalamus

The hypothalamus is involved in autonomic function and it also makes and releases hormones that help control and regulate body function. It is known to control motivational behaviours such as hunger and thirst and is involved in the body's natural circadian patterns of sleep and wakefulness. It also plays a role in the maintenance of body temperature.

Neurotransmission and the synapse

Neurotransmission is the process of electrical and chemical communication in the brain and central nervous system. Transmission of messages occurs between cells in the brain called neurons. Neurons vary in their appearance but all have a similar structure.

The neuron

- *Cell body* – each neuron has a cell body that consists of the main aspects of the cell, the nucleus, and cytoplasm and, in the case of neurons, the dendrites (Figure 5.2).
- *Axon* – the axon proceeds from the cell body and is long and thin. It can be surrounded by myelin, but not all are.
- *Axon terminal* – this is at the end of the axon and is where the nerve endings are found that make up the synapse with the next neuron dendrites.

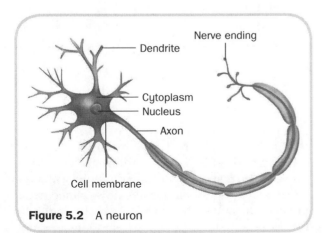

Figure 5.2 A neuron

The neuron or nerve cell is the main constituent of all brain tissue and responsible for coordination and communication. Nerve impulses pass down each neuron from the cell body, where the nucleus is contained, along the axon and down to the nerve endings where neurotransmission in the form of chemical communication between one nerve cell and another can then take place.

Receptors located on the dendrites in the cell body respond to a chemical message from another cell. This chemical message is converted to an electrical impulse that is conducted down the axon. Some axons are insulated with a substance called myelin that surrounds the axon and helps speed up electrical impulse transmission. The electrical impulse ends in the nerve terminal where it is converted into a chemical message ready for transmission across a synapse to the next neuron or point of communication.

The synapse

The synapse is a space between one neuron and another. This is where a chemical called a neurotransmitter is released from one neuron (pre-synaptic neuron) and can activate a receptor on a second neuron (post-synaptic neuron) to propagate neuronal transmission. These chemicals are monoamines and are stored in the neurons themselves, in vesicles ready for release once triggered by an electrical impulse. Once released into the synapse and after they have activated receptors they are taken back up into the pre-synaptic neuron either by passive diffusion or by means of a transporter. See if you can identify where the monoamines come from and go to in Figure 5.3. Some monoamines are broken down by enzymes in the synapse or nerve terminal called monoamine oxidases.

Monoamines and their roles

Monoamines are the chemicals in the brain involved in the process of neurotransmission outlined above. The main monoamines involved in neurotransmission are:

- 5-hydroxytryptamine (serotonin);
- acetylcholine;
- adrenaline;

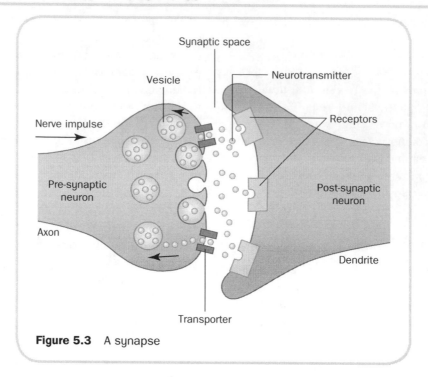

Figure 5.3 A synapse

- dopamine;
- gamma-aminobutyric acid (GABA);
- glutamate;
- noradrenaline;

Monoamines are specific to the neurons they are contained within and some are excitatory (these activate neurons or increase a response) whereas others are inhibitory (these deactivate neurons or reduce a response). Some neurotransmitters can possess excitatory and inhibitory action dependant not on the neurons they are in but the receptors they bind to after release.

5-hydroxytryptamine

More commonly known as serotonin, this neurotransmitter is involved in mood. It is found in the central nervous system but also in large amounts in the gut where it is involved in peristalsis, which is the movement of the gut. As well as being linked to mood and wellbeing it has functions in the regulation of appetite and plays a part in sleep patterns. Medications that act on serotonin systems are important in the management of mental health disorders related to these

functions. Serotonin has excitatory and inhibitory functions.

Acetylcholine

Acetylcholine is found in the central nervous system and in the periphery. It is a neurotransmitter in the classical sense but it also has actions in the brain that are neuromodulatory, that is, they are involved in the processing of information. Acetylcholine as a transmitter acts at many receptors including nicotinic and muscarinic receptors and it is excitatory in action. It is involved in memory, attention and decision making in the central nervous system as well as muscular movement in the periphery.

Adrenaline (epinephrine)

This neurotransmitter and hormone is found widely throughout the body and has many important functions. It is best known for its role in the 'fight or flight' response, whereby in stressful or life-threatening situations adrenaline is released in response to the situation, which increases heart rate and breaks down glycogen to glucose, to make the body 'ready' to deal with the situation. It is linked to emotions such as fear, and memory can be enhanced in fearful situations which may be due to the release of adrenaline. It has some links with PTSD due to this. It is excitatory in nature.

Dopamine

Dopamine is a neurotransmitter that has excitatory and inhibitory actions. It is found in the central nervous system and in the periphery. The main function in the brain is in the pleasure and reward pathways and is linked to motivation and addiction. It also has functions in motor control and the initiation of movement. There are many different dopamine receptors located in the brain and it is dependent on which type of receptor the dopamine acts on that controls whether its effect is excitatory or inhibitory. It is implicated in schizophrenia, where too much dopamine is seen, and dopamine depletion is a factor of Parkinson's disease.

Gamma-aminobutyric acid

This is the major inhibitory neurotransmitter in the central nervous system. It is widely distributed in the brain and is abundant in nature. It is involved in many functions including motor control, vision and sleep. It has been implicated in anxiety as well as being linked with epilepsy. Due to this, it is a target for drug action, as medications that act at GABA receptors show a good effect in these conditions.

Glutamate

This excitatory neurotransmitter is found in higher concentrations than any other in the brain and central nervous system. It predominantly acts on N-methyl-D-aspartate receptors and is involved in learning and memory. This transmitter is found in the hippocampus in great amounts. It is also a precursor for GABA.

Noradrenaline (norepinephrine)

Like adrenaline, this is an excitatory neurotransmitter but there is much more of this in the central nervous system than there is adrenaline. It is also released in response to stressful situations and is linked to anxiety and to concentration and attention.

The process of neurotransmission

This complicated electrical and chemical process begins with the initiation of the electrical signal within a neuron through the generation of an action potential (Figure 5.4). This is where the electrical potential of the nerve cell membrane changes. It involves the opening and closing of certain ion channels to trigger the event.

Before the action potential the nerve cell membrane is at its resting potential. Sodium channels open and sodium ions flow into the cell (1). This raises the membrane potential and depolarization occurs (2). Once peak action potential has been achieved the sodium channels close and the potassium channels then open, allowing potassium ions to flow out of the cell (the sodium ions are also being actively transported out of the cell) through the open channels causing the membrane potential to fall and repolarization then occurs (3). For a short time after an action potential the potassium channels stay open and hyperpolarization can occur (4) before the membrane returns to its resting potential (5).

This initiates the conduction of the electrical signal from the cell body, down the axon to the terminal area of the neuron where it is then converted from an electrical signal to a chemical signal by triggering the release of the neurotransmitter from the nerve ending into the synapse.

Understanding the basic structure and function of the brain regions, the synapses and

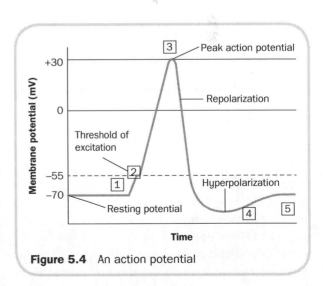

Figure 5.4 An action potential

the neurotransmitters involved will help you with understanding some of the altered physiology discussed in the subsequent chapters of this book. It will also allow you to grasp the pharmacological actions of many of the medications we will come on to discuss in the treatment and management of common mental health disorders.

Key learning points

Structure and function of the brain

▶ The nurse should be familiar with the main structures of the brain and the functions related to those structures.
▶ Some structures have many different functions: some motor, some sensory and some cognitive.

Neurotransmission and monoamines

▶ The nurse should be familiar with the concept of neurotransmission.
▶ The structure of the synapse and the neuron should be understood.
▶ You should be conversant with the different monoamines involved in neurotransmission and the process of nerve cell communication itself.

Multiple choice questions

Try answering these multiple choice questions to test what you have learned from reading this chapter. You can check your answers on page 151.

1 **What is the gap between two neurons where nerve transmission can occur called?**

   a) Synapse
   b) Terminal
   c) Junction
   d) Cell

2 **The neurotransmitter serotonin has which chemical name?**

   a) Dopamine
   b) Noradrenaline
   c) 5-hydroxytryptamine
   d) Adrenaline

3 **The hippocampal area of the brain is involved in what function?**

   a) Hormone production
   b) Breathing
   c) Movement
   d) Memory

$\longrightarrow$

←

4 GABA is the major _____ neurotransmitter in the brain?

a) Inhibitory
b) Excitatory
c) Classical
d) Glial

5 What is the bundle of tissue that connects the two hemispheres of the brain called?

a) Midbrain
b) Corpus callosum
c) Cerebellum
d) Cell body

6 The amygdala is part of the

a) Cerebellum
b) Brain stem
c) Spinal cord
d) Limbic system

7 How many lobes is the brain separated into?

a) 2
b) 4
c) 6
d) 8

8 Neurotransmitters are stored in nerve terminals in

a) The axon
b) Receptors
c) Vesicles
d) Glia

9 Myelin can surround what part of a neuron?

a) The axon
b) The nucleus
c) The cell body
d) The dendrites

10 What structure is known as the 'little brain'?

a) Cerebellum
b) Midbrain
c) Pons
d) Medulla

Recommended websites

http://www.brainfacts.org/
This website is a good starting point for brain basics for any learner.
http://www.brainline.org
This website allows you to find out the basics about traumatic brain injury and take an interactive journey through the brain to understand structure and function.

Recommended further reading

Waugh, A. & Grant, A. (2014) *Ross and Wilson Anatomy and Physiology in Health and Illness, 12th edn.* Oxford: Churchill Livingstone.

Anxiety disorders

6

Chapter contents

Learning objectives

Introduction

The classifications of anxiety disorder

The physiology of anxiety

Interventions in managing anxiety

The pharmacology of anxiolytic medication

Key learning points

Drug calculations

Multiple choice questions

Case studies

Recommended websites

Recommended further reading

Learning objectives

After reading this chapter you will have gained knowledge around:

■ The group of conditions categorized as anxiety disorders.

■ The physiology and pharmacology around each of the anxiety disorders.

■ The pharmacodynamic actions of drugs used in anxiety disorders.

Introduction

Anxiety is a perfectly normal and healthy emotion, most often experienced in situations of uncertainty or fear. Many of you reading this will have experienced feelings of anxiety in your lifetime and can relate to some of the symptoms that will be described. This does not mean that you are suffering from an anxiety disorder but that your life experiences are eliciting normal emotional responses that you cope with and learn from. But anxiety disorder occurs when this normal emotional response is experienced in ordinary, non-threatening situations or is felt continually, intolerably or in a disabling manner. There are many forms of anxiety disorder which will be discussed in this chapter, with generalized anxiety disorder (GAD) being the most common and therefore discussed in more detail.

The classifications of anxiety disorder

There are six main classifications of anxiety disorders:

- Panic disorder;
- Social phobia;
- GAD;
- Obsessive–compulsive disorder (OCD);
- Post-traumatic stress disorder (PTSD);
- Mixed anxiety and depressive disorder.

The definition of anxiety disorders can be found in section F40 and F41 of the ICD-10 Classification (WHO 2016). In section F40 a variety of anxiety disorders are broken down according to their causation, and this section covers agoraphobia, social phobias and specific (isolated) phobias. In section F41 the general anxiety disorders are addressed. These are panic attacks (episodic paroxysmal anxiety), GAD, and mixed anxiety and depression. All these conditions have a core set of symptoms that you will encounter, which are physical, emotional and psychological in nature. These are:

1. palpitations, pounding of the heart or an accelerated heart rate;
2. sweating;
3. trembling or shaking;
4. dry mouth (not associated with dehydration or medication);
5. difficulty breathing;
6. feelings of choking;
7. chest discomfort;
8. nausea or abdominal distress;
9. feeling dizzy, unsteady, faint or light-headed;
10. feeling that objects are unreal (derealization) or that one's self is distant or not really here (depersonalization);
11. fear of losing control, going crazy or passing out;
12. fear of dying;
13. hot flushes or cold chills;
14. numbness or tingling sensations.

As well as these symptoms there will often be a significant amount of emotional distress experienced by the patient due to the anxiety symptoms themselves or the avoidance of any recognized triggers. There may also be a recognition that the responses are excessive or unreasonable. These emotions can manifest as discomfort, fear, worry, rumination or continued business of thoughts around the anxiety focus. The sufferer may not be able to verbalize their emotions to you at this point but non-verbal communication by the healthcare professional is important to detect any visible signs of emotional anxiety or distress. In the definitions of the various conditions outlined below we will refer to this list as 'the list of common symptoms'.

Panic disorder

Panic attacks are characterized by the following:

- a discreet episode of intense fear or discomfort;
- abrupt onset;
- reaching a crescendo within a few minutes and lasting at least some minutes.

This is accompanied by at least four of the list of common symptoms at least one of which is from the first four symptoms on the list. They can happen in response to a trigger but often arise out of nowhere and for no apparent reason that can be detected by the patient or anyone with them.

Social phobia

Social phobia is defined as occurring when one of the following symptoms occur:

- marked fear of being the focus of attention, or fear of behaving in a way that would be embarrassing or humiliating;
- marked avoidance of being the focus of attention or situations where there is a fear of behaving in an embarrassing or humiliating way.

The definition also states that the patient should have at least two of the list of common symptoms one of which is from the first four symptoms on the list. This is suggestive of social phobia rather than just shy introverted behaviour.

These fears are manifested in situations like parties and meetings and can be heightened by eating in the presence of other people or the need to perform a task such as public speaking. Symptoms of social phobia may also include blushing, a fear of vomiting and an urge to micturate or defecate or the fear of needing to micturate or defecate. The symptoms are restricted to or predominant in the feared situation or when thinking about that situation.

Generalized anxiety disorder

GAD is defined as at least four of the list of common symptoms at least one of which is from the first four symptoms on the list. In this case the list of general symptoms is augmented by:

15. muscle tension or aches and pains;
16. restlessness and an inability to relax;
17. feeling 'keyed up' or on edge, or a feeling of mental tension;
18. a sensation of a lump in the throat or difficulty swallowing.

Also GAD is associated with:

- an exaggerated response to minor surprises or being startled;

- difficulty in concentrating;
- persistent irritability;
- difficulty getting to sleep.

It is the most common form of anxiety disorder and is often diagnosed as such because the anxiety does not fit into any other category of disorder we have looked at here but has enough of the core and ancillary symptoms to meet the criteria for diagnosis of anxiety.

Obsessive–compulsive disorder

This is classed with anxiety disorders as anxiety is almost always present. The condition is also characterized by obsessive thought patterns and by the person feeling compelled to perform certain acts. These thoughts and acts are recurrent and repetitive in nature. Some of the behaviour is often referred to as ritualistic in nature and the sufferer finds themselves unable to resist the acts and if they do resist severe anxiety is triggered.

Post-traumatic stress disorder

This anxiety related disorder is a response to a 'trauma' that has occurred in the past. The response can be after a few months but may be delayed for a longer period of time, even years after an event has occurred. The trauma does not need to have been physical and, indeed, it is often a stressful life event or series of events or an extreme situation. Sufferers describe flashbacks where they re-live the event or events that caused the emotional trauma. These can occur in sleep or when awake and can be triggered by surroundings or simply arise out of nowhere. Anxiety and depression are commonly associated with this condition.

Mixed anxiety and depressive disorder

We should also be aware that these symptoms commonly occur alongside depressive symptoms (see Chapter 7 for more on depression) in patients with a mixed anxiety and depressive disorder.

It is important that mental health nurses have a good understanding of the physiological mechanisms thought to be involved in anxiety disorders.

Although we do not have complete knowledge and understanding of the aetiology and pathophysiology involved, there is good evidence to support many theories around the development of anxiety and anxiety-related disorders. This knowledge allows for good understanding of how to ensure appropriate pharmacological and non-pharmacological treatment of the anxiety disorder in question.

The physiology of anxiety

Anxiety can be caused by many factors. Some can be said to be triggers for anxiety reactions, such as things that happen in our environment, substance misuse or stress, and others can be said to be endogenous factors, such as changes in brain chemistry or medical factors. Psychological factors also play a part as can personality traits such as low self-esteem and confidence. Many sufferers can in fact, without intention, make their anxiety state worse by worrying about it and therefore adding to the symptoms they are experiencing.

Anxiety is often a normal response to a situation, triggering a 'fight or flight' response in which the body prepares to protect or defend itself in stressful situations. Chemicals such as adrenaline and noradrenaline are involved. In a lot of stressful situations this can be useful and helpful and indeed some people admit to working well under pressure, probably due to the release of these chemicals and their physiological actions. But when the symptoms of anxiety are not seen to be linked to a trigger, or if linked, last longer and are more severe than would be reasonable from a trigger, or if they prevent someone from going about their normal life, then anxiety disorder can be diagnosed.

The neurotransmitters commonly involved in anxiety include:

- adrenaline;
- noradrenaline;
- GABA.

The involvement of these neurotransmitters in brain regions such as the amygdala and the hippocampus can help us to relate this to normal physiology, and its disruption can lead to the symptoms of anxiety listed near the beginning of this chapter. If it helps you, revise the chapter on anatomy and physiology of the brain to ensure you understand the mechanisms being discussed in this chapter.

This knowledge also helps us to understand how some of the medications used in the treatment and management of the symptoms of anxiety disorders might work. We will now come on to look at these in more detail.

Interventions in managing anxiety

Anxiety can be managed by pharmacological and non-pharmacological interventions, or a combination of the two. It is important that the patient is allowed to take a central role in the decision making with regard to treatment where appropriate. This will improve the adherence to any medication regime that may be initiated as well as forging a good patient–professional relationship based on mutual understanding and trust. It can also help to involve the patient's family or care support network in the plan of care. Many anxiety sufferers benefit from support groups or self-help material and this should be offered where it is prudent to do so.

Psychological therapies can be very helpful in the management of anxiety disorders and should be considered for all sufferers. These therapies can take many forms and some can be seen in Table 6.1.

The clinical guidelines produced by NICE provide clear, helpful guidance on medication use as part of anxiety management strategies. In particular you may want to become more familiar with the following (references and web links can be found at the end of the chapter).

- CG113: *Generalised Anxiety Disorder and Panic Disorder in Adults: Management* (NICE 2011).
- CG31: *Obsessive Compulsive Disorder and Body Dysmorphic Disorder: Treatment* (NICE 2005a).
- CG26: *Post-Traumatic Stress Disorder: Management* (NICE 2005b).

Table 6.1 Therapies available to help manage anxiety disorders

Therapy	Format
Cognitive–behavioural therapy (CBT)	One to one, face to face Online available
Relaxation techniques	One to one or group Self-help tools available
Meditation	One to one, group, face to face Online available Self-help tools available
Stress management	One to one, face to face Self-help tools available
Phobia therapy	One to one, face to face

■ CG159: *Social Anxiety Disorder: Recognition, Assessment and Treatment* (NICE 2013).

There are medications that can also be used to help manage the symptoms and manifestations of anxiety disorders and we will go on to examine the most common in the next part of this chapter.

The pharmacology of anxiolytic medication

Benzodiazepines

These drugs, despite their high addictive potential, remain very effective anxiolytics. The key to their proper use is safe and appropriate prescribing.

They act by potentiating the effect of GABA at its receptors in the central nervous system, thereby increasing its inhibitory neurotransmission effect in the brain. They bind to a benzodiazepine receptor located on the $GABA_A$ receptor and increase the likelihood of the ion channel opening. This occurs in the amygdala and limbic system in general. They have their anxiolytic effect at low dose but due to a development of tolerance often increasing doses are needed to maintain effect and long-term use is not recommended due to addiction potential. A main side-effect is sedation and this is related to the potentiation of nerve cell inhibition in firing. They can be used in treatment of acute anxiety or as a short-term solution while psychological therapy is being commenced. They may also be considered as an aid to sleep, but

again this should be for a short time only due to their propensity to cause addiction.

Antidepressants

Some of the antidepressant medications have been shown to have some benefit in anxiety disorders, with particular effect seen in GAD and mixed anxiety and depressive disorder.

The selective serotonin reuptake inhibitors

The selective serotonin reuptake inhibitors (SSRIs) commonly used in depressive disorders have been shown to be effective in treating some forms of anxiety disorder. Not all SSRIs are suitable for all anxiety disorders, however, and care should be used in selecting the correct drug at the correct dose once a firm diagnosis has been established. Doses of these drugs in anxiety management tend to be lower, certainly at initiation, than those seen in depression and should be titrated up slowly and in line with patient response. See Table 6.2 for commonly used SSRIs in anxiety disorders.

Another drug with SSRI action is venlafaxine, which also has action as a noradrenalin reuptake inhibitor and it can also be used in social phobia and GAD. The drug trazodone (a triazolopyridine antidepressant) can also be used, again at lower doses than in depression, for all forms of anxiety disorder.

The effects of these drugs in anxiety are thought to be similar in action to that of their antidepressant properties (outlined in more detail in

Table 6.2 Commonly used selective serotonin reuptake inhibitors (SSRIs) for anxiety disorders

SSRI	Anxiety disorder
Citalopram	Panic disorder
Escitalopram	Panic disorder Social phobia
Fluvoxamine	Obsessive–compulsive disorder (OCD)
Paroxetine	Social phobia Post-traumatic stress disorder (PTSD) Generalized anxiety disorder
Sertraline	Social phobia PTSD OCD

Chapter 7 on depressive disorders where these drugs are discussed in relation to their effect in their main area of prescribing).They are effective by increasing the amounts of neurotransmitters available in the synapse for action on receptors, but may also be linked to their ability to affect the fear response.

Tricyclic antidepressants

The tricyclic antidepressants (TCAs) would not be used in first-line management of anxiety, as we have better and safer drugs to use first, but they may be considered if a patient is not responding to other therapies. Clomipramine can be used in phobic and obsessional states but slow titration and close monitoring should be used.

Antipsychotics

Some drugs that are traditionally classed as antipsychotic medications have been used to manage some symptoms and manifestations of anxiety disorder. They are not a first-line choice of treatment and the use of them has been suggested as inappropriate by the NICE guidelines in 2011. The drug haloperidol has been used to manage agitation and anxiety in some patients.

Beta blockers

These are used to manage some of the physical symptoms that occur in anxiety such as palpitations, sweating, breathing difficulties and trembling. The drug propranolol is the most commonly

used example and is helpful in anxiety states where symptoms such as sweating, palpitations and tremor are problematic. The dose is lower than that which would be given of this drug when it is used for its primary purpose of treating high blood pressure, and a typical dose is 40mg once daily, increased to three times daily if needed to manage the symptoms. Patient blood pressure should be monitored to ensure that hypotension is not occurring.

Other drugs

Buspirone

This is an azapirone drug that has some action at serotonin receptors and has a license for short-term use in anxiety disorders. It can be given two to three times daily for the relief of anxiety and has been seen to have some effect on psychological symptoms such as poor concentration and irrational worry.

Pregabalin (Lyrica)

This drug is an anticonvulsant medication that has also been shown to be effective in the management of neuropathic pain and in GAD. Given orally in anxiety management it is given at a dose greater than seen in seizure management but equivalent to its dose in pain management. It can be titrated upwards if needed and this should be done at weekly intervals. Its effects in anxiety treatment are thought to be derived from its ability to bind to calcium channels in neurons and decrease their excitability thereby having an inhibitory effect.

Zopiclone

Zopiclone belongs to the group of drugs known as z-drugs used in the management of sleep disorders and insomnia. They can be useful, for short-term use only, in the management of anxiety where sleep deprivation is a significant problem. It is a cyclopyrrolone drug and has actions on the GABA system in the brain and central nervous system. It has a similar action to the benzodiazepines but is chemically unrelated and has some similar properties such as tolerance and addictive potential. Treatment is not recommended for longer than a four-week period as after use for longer than this time withdrawal signs can be seen upon stopping the medication.

It is important that you gain a working familiarity with these medications used in practice. You should be able to use the BNF to look up the medicines and to ascertain any effects and side-effects your patients may experience. You should also be able to use Appendix One of the BNF to check for interactions that these medications may have with other medications your patient may be taking at the same time.

Key learning points

Classifications of anxiety

▶ Anxiety is not one disorder but many disorders with similar symptoms.
▶ Symptoms can be physical, emotional or psychological.
▶ Correct diagnosis is essential so that pharmacological or non-pharmacological treatment can be initiated appropriately.

Physiology and pharmacology

▶ Medication can be used to manage physical and psychological symptoms.
▶ Some anxiolytic medication has addictive properties.
▶ Guidelines and the BNF should be used to assist in decision making around pharmacological treatment in anxiety disorders.
▶ Psychological therapies can be very valuable tools in the management of anxiety.

Drug calculations

1 Your patient requires 4mg of diazepam, four times per day. You have 2mg tablets.

How many tablets per dose?

How many tablets per day?

How many tablets for a 28-day supply?

2 Your patient requires 40mg of propranolol every 12 hours. You have 10mg tablets.

How many tablets per dose?

How many tablets per day?

How many tablets for a seven-day supply?

3 Your patient requires 15mg of buspirone twice daily. You have 5mg tablets.

How many tablets per dose?

How many tablets per day?

4 Your patient requires 7.5g of zopiclone at bedtime. You have 3.75mg tablets.

How many tablets per dose?

How many tablets for a 28-day supply?

5 Your patient requires 300mg of moclobemide twice daily. You have 150mg tablets.

How many tablets per dose?

How many tablets per day?

How many tablets for a 28-day supply?

6 Your patient requires clomipramine 25mg tablets daily for seven days, then twice daily for seven days, then 50mg daily (one dose) for seven days, then 50mg twice daily for seven days. You have 25mg tablets.

How many tablets for the 28-day supply?

7 Your patient requires trazodone 75mg daily. You have 50mg/5ml oral solution.

How many ml per day?

How much for a 28-day supply?

8 Your patient requires paroxetine 10mg daily. You have 2mg/ml oral suspension.

How many ml per day?

How much for a 28-day supply?

9 Your patient requires chlorpromazine 25mg three times a day for short-term use only. You have 5mg/ml solution.

How many ml per dose?

How many ml per day?

10 Your patient requires alprazolam 500 micrograms three times a day for short-term use only. You have 250 microgram tablets.

How many tablets per dose?

How many tablets per day?

Multiple choice questions

Try answering these multiple choice questions to test what you have learned from reading this chapter. You can check your answers on page 151.

1 What class of drugs does diazepam belong to?

a) Antidepressants
b) Benzodiazepines
c) Beta blockers
d) Hypnotics

2 What class of drugs does propranolol belong to?

a) Antidepressants
b) Benzodiazepines
c) Beta blockers
d) Hypnotics

3 What is the most common form of anxiety disorder?

a) Panic disorder
b) GAD
c) OCD
d) PTSD

4 Complete the sentence. Benzodiazepines can be addictive

a) But only when given with other anxiolytic drugs
b) Although not when the patient is told of the risks
c) But risks of addiction increase the more that it is used
d) But only at very high doses

5 The symptoms of anxiety can be

a) Physical
b) Emotional
c) Psychological
d) All of the above

6 What feature characterizes PTSD?

a) Anxiety
b) Depression
c) Flashbacks
d) Amnesia

7 What anxiety disorder can clomipramine be used in?

a) GAD
b) Phobia
c) PTSD
d) Mixed anxiety and depression

8 When can zopiclone be used in the management of anxiety?

a) If the patient requests it
b) If benzodiazepines are not suitable
c) If sleep is disturbed
d) If the patient has a phobia

9 What symptoms do beta blockers help with?

a) Physical
b) Emotional
c) Psychological
d) All of the above

10 What receptors do benzodiazepines act on?

a) Serotonin
b) Adrenaline
c) Noradrenaline
d) GABA

Case studies

(1) Mrs Lee is a 47-year-old married woman. She is the mother to two teenage boys who live at home. She has suffered from postnatal depression in the past and was successfully treated with fluoxetine. She now presents to the GP with the following symptoms and thinks she is depressed again:

- irritability;
- anxiety;
- poor sleep;
- appetite disturbance;
- agitations, palpitations and sweating;
- irrational fear-like feelings.

The GP does not diagnose depression. What do you think the diagnosis is and how might the treatment plan for Mrs Lee be formulated?

(2) James Jackson is 30 years old and has recently returned home to work after 12 years in the army. His last tour of duty was in Afghanistan where he lost four colleagues in a land vehicle attack where he was the only survivor. His symptoms are:

■ flashbacks to the attack – these seem real and he can see/hear and even smell what was around him at the time;

■ poor sleep;

■ social isolation and agoraphobia;

■ anger issues.

What is the likely diagnosis and course of treatment for James?

Recommended websites

British National Formulary (BNF): www.bnf.org
EMC medicines compendium: www.medicines.org.uk

Recommended further reading

National Institute for Health and Care Excellence (2005a) *Obsessive Compulsive Disorder and Body Dysmorphic Disorder: Treatment. CG31.* London: NICE. Available at: https://www.nice.org.uk/guidance/cg31 (accessed 22 February 2016).

National Institute for Health and Care Excellence (2005b) *Post-Traumatic Stress Disorder: Management. CG26.* London: NICE. Available at: https://www.nice.org.uk/guidance/cg26 (accessed 22 February 2016).

National Institute for Health and Care Excellence (2011) *Generalised Anxiety Disorder and Panic Disorder in Adults: Management. CG113.* London: NICE. Available at: https://www.nice.org.uk/guidance/cg113 (accessed 22 February 2016).

National Institute for Health and Care Excellence (2013) *Social Anxiety Disorder: Recognition, Assessment and Treatment. CG159.* London: NICE. Available at: https://www.nice.org.uk/guidance/cg159 (accessed 22 February 2016).

World Health Organization (WHO) (2016). *International Statistical Classification of Diseases and Related Health Problems 10th Revision (ICD-10) – WHO Version for 2016.* Available at: http://apps.who.int/classifications/icd10/browse/2016/en (accessed 19 February 2016).

Depressive disorders

7

Chapter contents

Learning objectives

After reading this chapter you will have gained knowledge around:

- The different manifestations of depressive disorder.
- The physiology and pharmacology of depressive disorder.
- The pharmacodynamic actions of drugs used in depressive disorders.

Introduction

Depression is a broad and heterogeneous diagnosis, with many differing 'layers' of depressed mood. It is, however, typically characterized by depressed mood and/or loss of pleasure in most activities. A definition of depression can be found in section F32 of the ICD-10 (WHO 2016). This lays out the various forms of depression and their definitions. However, there is a basic underlying diagnostic criteria for depressive illness as having at least two of the typical symptoms of depression with at least two of the other symptoms of depression. The duration of these symptoms should be at least two weeks. The 'typical' and 'other' symptoms of depression from the ICD-10 are listed and explained below.

Typical symptoms of depression
(main diagnostic symptoms):

- depressed or low mood;
- loss of or greatly reduced interest and enjoyment;
- increased fatigability (tire easily).

Other symptoms of depression (known as ancillary symptoms):

- reduced concentration and attention;
- reduced self-esteem and self-confidence;
- ideas of guilt and unworthiness (even in a mild episode);
- bleak and pessimistic views of the future (nihilism);
- ideas or acts of self-harm or suicide;
- disturbed sleep pattern;
- diminished appetite (but sometimes increased).

It is the intensity of these symptoms together with the number of symptoms present, and put together with other criteria, that we can use to gauge the severity of and therefore classify the depressive illness. Put simply, the more symptoms present and the more severe within the category, the worse the classification of depression.

There are a number of diagnostic tools that can be used to gauge the severity of a depressive episode and also to monitor any improvements or deteriorations seen in that illness in response to treatment. These would include the Patient Health Questionnaire (PHQ-9) originally designed and copyrighted by Pfizer and the Hospital Anxiety and Depression Scale (HADS) score. Different hospital trusts and different areas of practice will have their own preferences as to which tool they prefer. In view of this it may be worthwhile setting aside some time to refresh your knowledge of the local protocols in your area of practice with regard to this. These questionnaires are easy to find on the internet and are widely used.

The classifications of depressive disorder

Within this chapter we are only going to consider the features, management and pharmacological interventions in unipolar depression; for discussions around bipolar affective disorder (sometimes referred to as bipolar depression or an older term of manic depression) please see Chapter 10 of this textbook.

The National Institute for Health and Care Excellence base their definition of the severity of depression on the definitions used in the Diagnostic and Statistical Manual of Mental Disorders (DSM-IV, American Psychiatric Association 1994) and ICD-10 (WHO 2016). This leads to the following classifications for the severity of depression.

- *Subthreshold depressive symptoms*, where the patient has fewer than five of the symptoms of depression (can be called reactive sadness and may be in response to a life event).
- *Mild depression*, where the patient has five or slightly more than five of the symptoms of depression and displays only a mild functional impairment.
- *Moderate depression*, defined as simply being the stage between mild and severe depression where more than five symptoms are seen.
- *Severe depression*, where the patient has most of the symptoms of depression and also shows

a marked functional impairment. There is also the implication that psychotic features always indicate severe depression, but are not necessary for a diagnosis of severe depression to be made.

The physiology of depression

The actual aetiology and development of depressive disorders is not completely understood. The theories relating to the disorder suggest that there are many factors involved in the development of depression including psychological, genetic, hormonal and neurochemical.

Neurochemical factors – the monoamine hypothesis

This is one of the most widely held understandings as to why depression can develop and why it is an endogenous process and not simply a reaction to a sad or unhappy event. It is worth reminding yourself of the functions and process of neurotransmission in Chapter 5 before reading further.

The main monoamine neurotransmitters implicated in depressive illness and also the main three targeted with antidepressant medication are:

- 5-hydroxytryptamine (serotonin);
- noradrenaline;
- dopamine.

There is no solid evidence to suggest that any one of these is more responsible for depression than the others and in fact the aim is not to 'find' which one may be responsible in your patient but to acknowledge that all play a part and find the most useful medication for them by following guidelines and monitoring patient response to the medication where prescribed.

The monoamine hypothesis tells us that the normal circulating levels of these chemicals are *reduced* in depressive illness.

The monoamine theory could explain why:

- drugs that deplete monoamines are depressant, such as reserpine, methyldopa;

- drugs that increase availability of monoamines can improve mood in depressed patients, for example SSRIs, TCAs and monoamine oxidase inhibitors (MAOIs);
- The concentration of monoamines is reduced in the cerebrospinal fluid of depressed patients.

The monoamine theory could not explain why:

- drugs that increase availability of monoamines have no effect on mood in depressed patients, for example amphetamines, cocaine;
- some older antidepressants have no effect on monoamine systems, such as iprindole;
- there is a therapeutic delay of two weeks for the full effects of antidepressants to be seen.

The aim of many of the common antidepressant medications used is to *increase* the levels of monoamines.

Hormonal influences

In clinically depressed patients, research has shown that many of them have increased levels of cortisol, commonly referred to as the stress hormone, that can reduce back to more normal levels when the depression resolves or is successfully treated.

Some patients with hormonal conditions such as thyroid problems or Cushing's disease (hypercortisolism) or Addison's disease (hypoadrenalism) can often display depression as part of, or in conjunction with, their hormonal imbalance.

Hormones are part of the endocrine system that also has an effect on brain function. Disruption to any of the levels of these hormones can have an effect on brain neurochemistry and function, leading to signs and symptoms of depression.

Genetic factors

Many patients with depression will reveal on consultation that family members have also suffered from the condition. This does not mean that there is a direct genetic link but does raise the possibility. What may also be the case is that there is a familial trend. This is not so much related to genetics but to environmental influences, and gives rise to the concepts of and debate around 'nature and nurture'. 'Nature' would relate to genetic links, and twin studies (commonly used in genetic determination of relationships in conditions) where identical twins who have been raised apart show an increased incidence of depression affecting both twins. 'Nurture' would relate to the family environment and upbringing and where twins have been raised together; in this situation there is an even higher incidence of depression affecting both twins.

Psychological factors

There are other factors that can play a part in the development of true depressive illness. Many patients have traits that can be seen to predispose them to depression as they are in fact some of the criteria for diagnosis. An example would be people with low self-esteem. On its own this is not sufficient to diagnose depression, but may be a triggering factor for other symptoms. It is also acknowledged that patients who suffer from anxiety can go on to develop depression (known as mixed disorder) if the anxiety is not managed. Other factors that may be contributory are:

- perfectionism;
- low levels of social support and isolation (sometimes loneliness is cited);
- major life events such as bereavement or stressful events or a significant medical diagnosis (see below);
- sleep disorders.

Other medical conditions

As outlined above, some conditions such as Cushing's and Addison's disease can predispose a person to depression. These are related to hormonal imbalances but other medical conditions can have an effect on mood to the extent that depression is precipitated. Long-term chronic conditions, by the nature of the diagnosis and the lifetime duration, can precipitate low mood leading to depression. This can also be true of cancer diagnosis, where the severity of the disease has such an effect

that depression is triggered. Parkinson's disease, where there is an imbalance of dopamine in the brain and central nervous system is also recognized as a common disorder where depression is possible.

Other medications

Certain medications which are given for other conditions have been implicated in depressive illness development. As you can see from some of the conditions above, if we give medications that are likely to affect monoamines or hormones within the body, then these drugs themselves may be triggers for chemical or hormonal imbalance leading to depression.

These include:

- corticosteroids;
- Parkinson's drugs;
- drugs used in anxiety and sleep disorder.

There are other drugs with no direct effect on steroids in the body or monoamines in the brain but depression has been recognized as a side-effect and these can be seen in the relevant sections of the BNF.

They include:

- pain relieving medications (many but specifically opioid analgesics);
- some anticonvulsant medications;
- some antihypertensive drugs;
- oral contraceptives.

It is worthwhile looking at medications your patients may be receiving and familiarizing yourself with some of the side-effects to see if depression is listed.

Interventions in managing depression

Once a diagnosis has been established, NICE guidance (CG90 and 91, NICE 2009a, 2009b) suggests a stepped model of care should be applied, where the treatment options are proportionate to the severity of the depression. This model would take the following form.

Step 1

■ For use with all known or suspected presentations of depression.

■ Assessment, support, psychoeducation, active monitoring and referral on for further assessment and interventions.

Step 2

■ Where there is persistent subthreshold depression or mild to moderate depression.

■ In these cases the options would include low-intensity psychological interventions, psychological interventions, medication and referral for further assessment and interventions.

Step 3

■ Where there is persistent subthreshold depression, or mild to moderate depression that has not responded to initial interventions, or moderate and severe depression.

■ Here the management options include medication, high-intensity psychological interventions, combined treatments, collaborative care and referral on to specialist services.

Step 4

■ Where there is severe and/or complex depression, where there may be a risk to life or a risk of severe self-neglect.

■ In these circumstances the model suggests treatment options should include medication, high-intensity psychological interventions, electroconvulsive therapy, crisis services intervention, combined treatments and multidisciplinary and/or inpatient care.

The take home message from this stepwise approach is that the treatment of depression is not simply pharmacological. There should be a holistic approach to the patient that includes talking therapies and active support as well as medication where appropriate. There is evidence that patients treated with this holistic approach have better outcomes that those treated with medication alone.

National Institute for Health and Care Excellence guidance on drug treatment (CG90 and 91)

This guidance (NICE 2009a, 2009b) suggests that there is no convincing evidence to suggest that the severity of the depression, the gender of the patient or their ethnicity need be taken into account when considering the drug treatment options available to the individual. There is evidence, however, that patients with severe concomitant disease should be approached in a more structured manner and we will consider this later in this chapter. It is important at this stage to point out that the guidance outlined here is for the treatment of the adult patient. The National Institute for Health and Care Excellence has not come up with a rigid protocol for the treatment of depression, rather they have emphasized the need to tailor treatment to the individual. Guidance is given, however, as to what to consider when tailoring the treatment to the individual.

The guidelines from NICE suggest that treatment should be initiated with an SSRI as they are regarded as being as effective as any other class of antidepressant while also having a more favourable side-effect profile than the other classes. This means that these drugs have lower risks associated with them and are seen as a safer medication. You should, however, be aware that no drug is completely safe and you must always use the BNF to check for side-effects, cautions and interactions with other medication.

If an SSRI is seen as unsuited to the patient, NICE suggests the use of other medication. The use of TCAs, with the exception of lofepramine, is associated with a greater risk of overdose and this is one of the main reasons for them being prescribed less often for depressive disorder today. The initiation of treatment with the non-reversible MAOIs should normally be limited to specialist mental health professionals and again these are being prescribed less often due to the availability of safer medications.

Initiation

When initiating medication the prescriber should start by discussing the choices of medication available and their potential adverse side-effects, the potential interactions with the other medications the patient may be on and the effects that the antidepressant medication may have on pre-existing disease processes. This discussion should also take into consideration the patient's previous experiences with antidepressant medications.

Explore the patient's concerns about medications and explain why you feel medication is needed. Give information about how the medication works. Explain that the full antidepressant effect may take a while to develop. Emphasize the need to take the medication as prescribed and to continue with the treatment even after remission has been achieved. Outline the possible side-effects and interactions of the medication. Also outline the potential risks and associated symptoms of withdrawing the medication in an uncontrolled fashion. It is important to stress the non-addictive nature of most of the antidepressant medications as, anecdotally, there appears to be a strong misconception in the mind of the general public with regard to this.

Monitoring

After initiating therapy, monitoring the patient's progress becomes paramount. For patients not deemed to be at risk of suicide NICE recommends initial review at two weeks after the initialization of treatment. Then it is suggested that regular review at an interval of every two to four weeks be carried out until three months after the initiation of therapy. After three months, if there has been a good response to treatment and the patient is stable, the interval between reviews may be extended further. If there is a perceived suicide risk the reviews should be weekly initially and more frequent thereafter. There is an increased prevalence of suicidal thought in the under-30 age group and this can be exacerbated by the initiation of antidepressant therapy. In view of this these patients should be treated as if they are at risk of suicide and reviewed accordingly.

Patients may develop side-effects in the early stages of treatment that resolve as treatment continues. The guidelines by NICE recommend the provision of written information about these potential effects. It also recommends that side-effects should be monitored closely and if they are mild and easily tolerated treatment should continue. However, the patient's perception of the severity of the side-effects should be considered and if necessary the medication should be stopped and an alternative antidepressant should be started. Consider the use of concomitant therapies that might alleviate the side-effects. For example, consider the use of benzodiazepines in the short term to help with any anxiety, agitation or insomnia symptoms that might occur. The guidance from NICE recommends that the use of these drugs should be limited in duration to no more than two weeks in view of their addictive nature.

If there is a limited or no response to treatment after two to four weeks NICE suggests checking patient compliance. If they are compliant and a therapeutic dose is in use it is suggested that the dose be increased if there is scope to do so or that another therapeutic agent is tried. When doing this, take into account the side-effects the patient is experiencing and the patient's preference. Use a validated assessment tool such as the PHQ-9 or HADS tools to document the patient's progress.

The use of combinations of drugs in the treatment of depression should only be considered after discussion with a consultant psychiatrist. This would include the use of adjunctive therapies such as lithium, olanzapine, quetiapine, mirtazapine and mianserin.

Continuation of therapy in remission

Once remission has been achieved NICE advise that drug therapy should be continued for six months in the first instance. This may need to be extended in patients who have a history of recurrent bouts of depression or who have persistent residual symptoms, concomitant physical health problems or psychosocial problems. In patients with a significant risk of recurrence then therapy should be continued for at least two years at the dose that produced the initial improvements while the patient was in the acute phase of their illness.

Withdrawal of therapy

When the time comes to stop treatment, NICE recommends that the patient is made aware of the potential withdrawal symptoms. Discontinuation should be done gradually with the dose being reduced slowly over a four-week period to lessen the risk of withdrawal symptoms. There is particular risk of developing these symptoms with the antidepressants with shorter half-lives (see Glossary), such as paroxetine or venlafaxine. This strategy of gradual dose reduction is not needed in patients stopping fluoxetine, however, because of its prolonged half-life. It is important to remind the patient to seek urgent review if they start to experience withdrawal effects. If this happens then the medication should be reintroduced at the therapeutic dose and the process of gradual withdrawal recommenced.

The guidance from NICE chooses to consider depression in adults with concomitant chronic physical disease as a separate problem (NICE 2009b). However, there is a lot of overlap between the two sets of guidance. It is estimated that the prevalence of depression in those suffering with a chronic physical disease is two to three times greater than that seen in the general population. In view of this NICE recommend that patients with chronic physical illness should be screened regularly to facilitate the early diagnosis and treatment of any depression that might occur. The guidance recommends the use of the following screening questions (NICE 2009b: p. 8).

■ During the last month, have you often been bothered by feeling down, depressed or hopeless?
■ During the last month, have you often been bothered by having little interest or pleasure in doing things?

If the patient answers 'yes' to either or both of these questions, NICE recommends further assessment is carried out to establish a more accurate understanding of the patient's condition prior to looking at potential interventions. The interventions recommended are dependent on the severity of the depression and are set out according to the stepped

model of care outlined above. Again this puts an emphasis on the holistic approach to the patient and recommends the use of talking therapies as well as drug-based interventions. However, there are specific issues around antidepressant use in the chronically physically ill that need to be considered.

Pharmacology of antidepressant medication

There are a few different categories of antidepressant medication, as mentioned above that we need to consider when we think about the pharmacology of drugs used to treat depression. These are outlined in Table 7.1 and are how antidepressants are classified in the BNF.

So we can now go on to look at the pharmacological actions of each of these classes of antidepressant drug.

Tricyclic antidepressants and related antidepressants

The TCAs are powerful antidepressants and have been around for many years. These drugs block the reuptake of two major monoamines, noradrenaline and serotonin, also known as 5-hydroxytryptamine. This means that there is more of the monoamine available in the synapse to act at the receptors and this has an antidepressant effect by enhancing neurotransmission. However, drugs in this class, such as amitriptyline, act at other receptors, which can lead to side-effects. The main side-effects are as follows.

■ Sedation. This can be useful if the drug is taken at night and insomnia is a problem. It can be increased if the drugs are taken with alcohol and this can be problematic.
■ Cardiac rhythm problems that can be severe in overdose.
■ Anticholinergic effects produced by action at muscarinic receptors, such as urinary retention and constipation.
■ These drugs can cause patients with epilepsy to have more seizures.

These side-effects mean that these drugs are not the first-line choice of treatment due to the

Table 7.1 **Antidepressant drugs**

Group	Abbreviation	Example
Tricyclic antidepressants	TCAs	Amitriptyline
Antidepressants related to TCAs		Trazodone
Monoamine oxidase inhibitors	MAOIs	Phenelzine
Reversible inhibitor of monamine oxidase A	RIMA	Moclobemide
Selective serotonin reuptake inhibitors	SSRIs	Sertraline Citalopram
Other drugs: Noradrenaline reuptake inhibitors Serotonin noradrenergic reuptake inhibitors Alpha adrenoceptor antagonists	NARIs SNRIs AAAs	Reboxetine Venlafaxine Mirtazapine

problems they can cause. They also are very toxic in overdose and this is particularly important to know if your depressed patient has thoughts of suicide.

Monoamine oxidase inhibitors

Monoamine oxidase exists in two forms, monoamine oxidase A and monoamine oxidase B, and they are responsible for chemically breaking down monoamines involved in neurotransmission that we have outlined above, to render them inactive. They are found in all neurons in the brain and central nervous system that produce monoamines. Drugs that block this breakdown are called MAOIs and phenelzine is an example. The blocking of this breakdown leads to an increase in the availability of the monoamines for neurotransmission which, like TCAs, leads to an antidepressant effect by increased receptor activation. This is represented in Figure 7.1.

These drugs are used infrequently now due to their high risk of drug interactions especially with other antidepressants. They are also able to interact negatively with some foodstuffs containing tyramine and dopamine (such as some cheeses, red wine, pickled herring and others). The interaction can lead to increased blood pressure up to a dangerous level and so patients on these medications are warned to avoid these foods. These drugs bind irreversibly but there is a reversible MAOI, moclobemide, which is also used. Specialist initiation and monitoring is required.

Selective serotonin reuptake inhibitors

The SSRIs act selectively at serotonin (5-hydroxy-tryptamine) neurons to produce their anti-depressant effect. They have very similar profiles

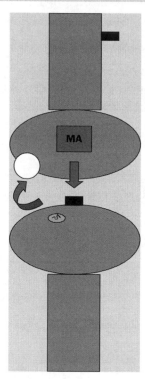

Figure 7.1 Monoamine (MA) transmission and oxidation. Key: neurons are in dark grey; the arrow dictates the route of release and reuptake of MA; the black boxes are the receptors; the clear circle represents the reuptake system; the light grey oval is monoamine oxidase.

regarding their antidepressant effects. The main differences between them lie with their abilities to cause drug interactions and effects and this is often the reason for choosing one over another in particular patients.

Serotonin is released from the neuron into the synapse to have its action upon receptors. After release it is taken back up into the neuron that released it by a transporter located in the neuronal membrane. The SSRIs inhibit the reuptake of serotonin from the synapse after it has been released. This leads to an increase in the amount present in the synapse and available for action at receptors, which respond to it enhancing neurotransmission. This has an antidepressant effect. Figure 7.2 shows the various parts involved.

The SSRIs have far fewer side-effects than other antidepressants and are safe in overdose. This makes them a good first-line choice of drug for treating most depressions. The main drugs prescribed in this class are sertraline and citalopram although escitalopram and fluoxetine are also seen. The main reported side-effects include nausea and diarrhoea, loss of sexual desire and libido, some anxiety during initiation of treatment and occasionally sleep disturbances.

The effects of SSRIs take up to 14 days to fully develop and this should be explained to patients at commencement of treatment.

Other drugs

There are some other drugs that are useful in the treatment of depression. They include the following.

- Mirtazapine – an alpha adrenoceptor antagonist that is a mildly sedating antidepressant.
- Reboxetine – a noradrenaline specific reuptake inhibitor (NARI).
- Venlafaxine – a noradrenaline and 5-hydroxytryptamine specific reuptake inhibitor that may have a quicker onset of action compared with noradrenaline or serotonin reuptake inhibitors alone.
- Tryptophan – this is a naturally occurring precursor to 5-hydroxytryptamine that is obtained

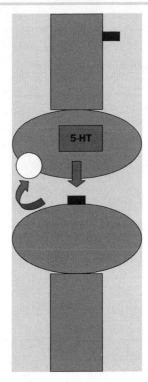

Figure 7.2   Serotonin (5-hydroxytryptamine, 5-HT) release and reuptake. Key: neurons are in dark grey; arrows dictate route of release and reuptake of 5-HT; black boxes are receptors; the clear circle is the reuptake system.

from our diet but can be given in its pure form. The theory is that if more of the precursor is available the body will make more 5-hydroxytryptamine leading to an antidepressant effect. It can be used as an adjunct therapy with MAOIs and TCAs.

It is important that you gain a working familiarity with these medications used in practice. You should be able to use the BNF to look up the medicines and to ascertain any effects and side-effects your patients may experience. You should also be able to use Appendix One of the BNF to check for interactions that these medications may have with other medications your patient may be taking at the same time.

Key learning points

Classifications of depression

▶ The nurse should be aware of the different classifications of depression and how interventions are targeted dependent on diagnosis.

▶ Depression may present in many ways and can be mild, moderate or severe.

Physiology and pharmacology

▶ The nurse should be aware of the physiological causes of and triggers for depressive disorder and be able to identify conditions and medications that may be linked to depression development.

▶ The nurse should be aware of the range of medications that can be used to treat or manage depression and the pharmacological actions of these drugs.

▶ The BNF is a good source of information about medications that are prescribed in depressive disorders with regards to effects, side-effects and interactions.

▶ Pharmacological treatment of depression is indicated in guidelines for depression that is moderate or severe in nature.

Drug calculations

1 Your patient is prescribed citalopram 40mg daily. You have 20mg tablets.

How many tablets per dose and for a 28-day supply?

2 Your patient is prescribed sertraline 150mg daily. You have 50mg tablets.

How many tablets per dose and for a 28-day supply?

3 Your patient is prescribed venlafaxine 300mg daily in TWO divided doses. You have 75mg tablets.

How many tablets per dose, per day and for a 28-day supply?

4 Your patient is prescribed mirtazapine 30mg at bedtime. You have 15mg tablets.

How many tablets per dose and for a 28-day supply?

5 Your patient is prescribed trazodone 300mg daily in THREE divided doses. You have 50mg capsules.

How many capsules per dose, per day and for a 28-day supply?

6 Your patient is prescribed lofepramine 210mg daily in TWO divided doses. You have 70mg in 5ml liquid.

How many ml per dose, per day and for a 28-day supply?

7 Your patient is prescribed moclobemide 300mg twice daily. You have 150mg tablets.

How many tablets per dose, per day and for a 28-day supply? ⟶

8 Your patient is prescribed escitalopram 10mg daily. You have 1mg/drop (20mg/ml) oral drops.

How many drops per day?

How many days will a 15ml bottle last?

9 Your patient is prescribed reboxetine 4mg twice daily for three weeks then 6mg twice daily for the fourth week. You have 4mg scored tablets.

How many tablets per dose and per day for weeks one to three?

How many tablets per dose and per day for week four?

How many tablets for the 28-day supply?

10 Your patient is prescribed fluoxetine 40mg daily. You have 20mg in 5ml solution.

How many ml per day and for a 28-day supply?

Multiple choice questions

Try answering these multiple choice questions to test what you have learned from reading this chapter. You can check your answers on page 152.

1 Citalopram belongs to which class of drugs?

   a) TCAs
   b) SSRIs
   c) NARIs
   d) MAOIs

2 What is the first-line treatment for mild depression?

   a) SSRIs
   b) Talking therapies
   c) MAOIs
   d) Electroconvulsive therapy

3 How long after initiation of antidepressant therapy should the patient be reviewed for effect?

   a) 3 months
   b) 1 month
   c) 2–4 weeks
   d) 1 week

$\longrightarrow$

4 SSRIs act on the re-uptake mechanism for which monoamine?

a) 5-hydroxytryptamine
b) Noradrenaline
c) Adrenaline
d) Dopamine

5 Moclobemide is an example of which class of antidepressant?

a) TCAs
b) SSRIs
c) NARIs
d) MAOIs

6 Once remission has been achieved, NICE advice is that drug therapy should be continued for

a) 1 month
b) 3 months
c) 6 months
d) 12 months

7 What are the numbers of the NICE clinical guidelines dealing with depression?

a) CG90/91
b) CG91/92
c) CG95/97
d) CG98/99

8 Step 4 of the NICE management guidelines is where the depression is

a) Mild
b) Mild to moderate
c) Moderate
d) Severe

9 Which of the following monoamines is implicated in depression?

a) Serotonin
b) Noradrenaline
c) Dopamine
d) All of the above

10 One of the main symptoms used to diagnose depression is

a) Raised blood pressure
b) Depressed or low mood
c) Poor sleep
d) Suicide attempt

Case study

Susan Jones is a 44-year-old woman with a history of recurrent depression that has been successfully managed in the past with SSRIs. She has attended for CBT before and found it helpful. She has been 'well' for five years but presents with:

- low mood;
- trouble getting to sleep and early morning waking;
- poor concentration;
- feelings of worthlessness;
- seeing 'no future' for herself.

She admits to thoughts of ending her life. According to the ICD-10 classification Susan is *moderately* depressed.

Outline how you as the prescriber may initiate treatments and management according to guidelines and how you as the nurse can be involved in the early stages of Susan's care.

Recommended websites

British National Formulary (BNF): www.bnf.org
EMC medicines compendium: www.medicines.org.uk

Recommended further reading

American Psychiatric Association (1994). *Diagnostic and Statistical Manual of Mental Disorder (4th edn) (DSM-IV)*. APA, 1994.

National Institute for Health and Care Excellence (2009a) *Depression in Adults: Recognition and Management. CG90*. London: NICE. Available at: https://www.nice.org.uk/guidance/cg90 (accessed 22 February 2016).

National Institute for Health and Care Excellence (2009b) *Depression in Adults with a Chronic Physical Health Problem: Recognition and Management. CG91*. London: NICE. Available at: https://www.nice.org.uk/guidance/cg91 (accessed 22 February 2016).

World Health Organization (WHO) (2016) *International Statistical Classification of Diseases and Related Health Problems 10th Revision (ICD-10) – WHO Version for 2016*. Available at: http://apps.who.int/classifications/icd10/browse/2016/en (accessed 19 February 2016).

Psychosis

Chapter contents

Learning objectives

Introduction

The classifications of psychosis

The physiology of psychosis

Interventions in managing psychosis

Pharmacology of antipsychotic medication

Key learning points

Drug calculations

Multiple choice questions

Case study

Recommended websites

Recommended further reading

Learning objectives

After reading this chapter you will have gained knowledge around:

- The conditions categorized as psychosis.
- The physiology and pharmacology around psychosis.
- The pharmacodynamic actions of drugs used as antipsychotics.

Introduction

The group of conditions known as the psychotic disorders will make up a significant proportion of the mental health disorders and patients that you will come across in your time as a mental health nurse. This chapter covers schizophrenic disorders and other disorders that fall into the category of psychosis. We will again be using the ICD-10 criteria (WHO 2016) to guide our classification and understanding of psychotic disorders before moving on to look at the physiological features of the conditions and the pharmacological interventions we can use to manage these conditions. The main feature of this group of conditions is the extreme disorder of thought and perception that is seen. Behaviour is very often bizarre and strange and emotions can be blunted. The time course and ultimate severity of the conditions varies from person to person and this can also be unpredictable in nature.

The classifications of psychosis

Strictly speaking there are no absolute diagnostic criteria for this condition, although there are a number of strongly associated symptoms that are highly suggestive. These have been broken down into nine groups of related symptoms.

1. Symptoms related to the manipulation of thoughts such as thought echo, thought insertion, thought withdrawal and thought broadcasting.

2. Delusions of control or influence. This may be applied to limb movements, actions or sensations, but may also be applied to thoughts and perceptions if delusional also.

3. Auditory hallucinations, specifically voices. These voices may be single or multiple. They may be giving a running commentary on the person's actions or discussing the individual among themselves. These voices may be felt to come from outside the body or from within. When felt to come from within they may appear to come from any part of the body.

4. Persistent delusions that are culturally inappropriate or impossible. These may include religiously or politically significant identities and superhuman powers or abilities.

5. Persistent hallucinations of any type when associated with delusional or persistently over-valued ideas. Also if these hallucinations occur daily and persist over weeks or months.

6. A break down in the chain of thought resulting in incoherent or irrelevant speech or the formation of neologisms

7. Catatonic behaviour including excitement, posturing, waxy flexibility, mutism or stupor.

8. So called negative symptoms such as apathy, reduced speech and blunting of affect. These are associated with social withdrawal and reduced social functioning. However, it also has to be certain that these negative symptoms do not relate to a depressive illness.

9. A significant and consistent change in the quality of personal behaviour. This can be seen as a loss of interest in things, idleness or aimlessness. It might also manifest as a self-absorbed attitude and social withdrawal.

The usual diagnostic guidance for schizophrenia suggests that the patient should have one clear symptom and at least two less clear-cut symptoms from the first four groups listed above. Alternatively patients should have symptoms from groups five to eight that are recognized as being present for most days over a period of one month or more. Symptoms in group nine apply only to simple schizophrenia and must be persistent for at least one year before a diagnosis can be made.

It is important to remember that the diagnosis of schizophrenia should not be made if there are symptoms strongly suggestive of depression or mania – unless the schizophrenic symptoms predate these. Schizophrenia should not be diagnosed if there is intracranial pathology such as significant head injury, space occupying lesions, epilepsy, treated Parkinson's disease or surgical trauma to the brain. Drug intoxication or withdrawal should also be excluded prior to diagnosis as some recreational drugs and alcohol can produce effects that mimic some of the symptoms of psychosis.

We will start by looking at the types of psychosis you are likely to encounter before we move on to look at the physiological aspects of psychosis.

Paranoid schizophrenia

This is the commonest form of the condition and is found in F20.0 of the ICD-10 classification (WHO 2016). Clinically it presents as a relatively stable condition, usually with the person having paranoid delusional ideas. It is also characterized by, and associated with, auditory hallucinations and disturbances in perception. The commonest paranoid symptoms can be broken into three types.

1. Delusions of persecution, reference, high-status birth, special mission, body change or jealousy.

2. Auditory hallucinations that may take the form of voices that are threatening or commanding. These may also take the form of whistling or laughing.

3. Hallucinations of the other sensory faculties, such as smell and sensation of touch although visual hallucinations are rare.

Thought disorder may also occur but it does not affect the ability to describe the hallucinations or delusions. Affect is usually less altered, although there may be mood disturbances and a degree of inappropriateness may be noted. Negative symptoms may be seen but tend not to be dominant.

Diagnosis is made using the system laid out above, although the emphasis is on the delusional and hallucinatory symptoms and the symptoms associated with disturbances in speech, affect, volition and movement are less noticeable.

Hebephrenic schizophrenia

This is a form of the disease in which changes in affect or mood predominate. It is seen under section F20.1 of the ICD-10 classification (WHO 2016). Delusions and hallucinations may be present but are usually short lived and fragmentary and the patient often behaves irresponsibly and unpredictably. The mood is often inappropriate and might manifest as giggling or a self-satisfied, self-absorbed smiling. Mannerisms are common, as are repeated phrases, hypochondriasis and pranks. Thought is disorganized and speech can be incoherent. The individual tends to be solitary and have little in the way of drive or motivation. A preoccupation with abstract thinking like religion or philosophy may be noticeable. The onset tends to be between the ages of 15 and 25 and there is a premorbid tendency towards shyness and solitude. This can initially be missed due to many changes in behaviour that are normal in the teenage years. There can be a rapid progression of the condition with the development of negative symptoms becoming predominant as time goes on.

Diagnosis is made using the system laid out above, although diagnosis for the first time should be made only in the appropriate age group with time given for normal adolescent quirks of behaviour to be ruled out. Often diagnosis will require several months of observation to ensure the characteristic behaviours are sustained and progressive.

Catatonic schizophrenia

Psychomotor disturbance is the main feature of this type of psychosis. It is seen under section F20.2 of the ICD-10 classification (WHO 2016). These disturbances can swing from hyperkinesia to stupor or anything in between. Constrained positions over prolonged periods of time may also be a feature, as may periods of violent excitement. This condition is less common in industrialized societies, although the reason for this is unknown. The catatonia may be associated with vivid, dreamlike, scenic hallucinations.

Diagnosis is made using the system laid out above, although the clinical picture will be predominated by one or more of the following features.

1. Stupor or mutism.
2. Excitement.
3. Posturing.
4. Negativism.
5. Rigidity.

6   Waxy flexibility – decreased response to stimuli and tendency to immobility.

7   Command automatism – aimless undirected behaviour.

Undifferentiated schizophrenia

This is where the diagnostic criteria laid out above are fulfilled, but there are no features to allow diagnostic differentiation into a clinical subgroup. It is described under section F20.3 of the ICD-10 classification (WHO 2016). It is also the case that there may be features associated with a number of the subgroups but no predominate feature manifests. It has also been referred to as atypical schizophrenia.

Post-schizophrenic depression

This is diagnosed as a normal depressive episode, which may be prolonged, but its onset comes after a noted schizophrenic episode. It is seen under section F20.4 of the ICD-10 classification (WHO 2016). There may be residual features of schizophrenia noted and these features may be positive or negative, although the negative features are commoner. It is not necessary to distinguish between depressive illnesses that started after the schizophrenic episode had settled or for it to have been a feature of the original illness. Although the depression rarely becomes severe there is an increased suicide risk associated with this condition.

Diagnosis can only be made if the patient has had a schizophrenic illness, some of those symptoms persist and the depressive symptoms become predominant and distressing.

Residual schizophrenia

A chronic stage of schizophrenia in which there is an obvious progression from the early stages of the disease to a more negative, long-term, although not always irreversible, illness. It is seen under section F20.5 of the ICD-10 classification (WHO 2016). Manifestations of this include dullness of mood, passivity in speech and behaviour, poor non-verbal communication and a deterioration in self-care.

Simple schizophrenia

This is uncommon and is outlined in section F20.6 of the ICD-10 classification (WHO 2016). It is characterized by the insidious onset and progression of oddities of behaviour, inability to meet the demands of society and a decline in function. Delusions and hallucinations are not common and there are none of the florid symptoms associated with the other subtypes of the disease. This makes diagnosis a real challenge and requires prolonged observation. Many people see this behaviour more as eccentricity rather than a mental health disorder.

Schizotypal disorder

Schizotypal disorder is elucidated in section F21 of the ICD-10 classification (WHO 2016). This condition is characterized by abnormalities in behaviour and thinking that resemble those seen in schizophrenia without any of these reaching the point of fulfilling the diagnostic criteria outlined above. There may be lapses into more psychotic phases. There is a tendency that the patients have relatives with full-blown schizophrenia and it might be that schizotypal disorder may represent a stage on a genetic spectrum for schizophrenia. It has also been called latent schizophrenia.

Acute and transient psychotic disorders

This continues to be a grey area and cannot be easily defined. They are considered in section F23 of the ICD-10 classification (WHO 2016). In view of this an order of priority has been defined for the symptoms.

1   An acute onset (within the last two weeks).

2   The presence of typical syndromes (outlined below).

3   The presence of an associated acute stress.

The typical syndromes are as follows.

1   Acute polymorphic psychotic disorder without symptoms of schizophrenia. Here there may be hallucinations, delusions and perceptual disturbances, but they are varied, changing

from day to day and even hour to hour. This disorder is particularly likely to have a sudden onset and a rapid resolution and in most cases there is no obvious precipitating stressor.

2 Acute polymorphic psychotic disorder with symptoms of schizophrenia. This is the same as above, but with symptoms of schizophrenia. This must have lasted at least one month and the variability may be present but is not as marked as it is in (1) above.

3 Acute schizophrenia-like psychotic disorder. Here the symptoms of schizophrenia are comparatively stable, but are short lived, lasting no more than one month.

4 Other acute predominantly delusional psychotic disorder. This is an acute disorder with comparatively stable delusions or hallucinations as its main feature. The delusions are usually of persecution or reference and the hallucinations are usually auditory where the voice talks directly to the patient.

Schizoaffective disorder

In this condition both affective and schizophrenic features may predominate at any one point within the same episode of illness. This may be simultaneously or within a few days of each other. There are three basic types outlined in section F25 of the ICD10 classification (WHO 2016).

1 Manic type. Here both schizophrenic and manic symptoms coexist within the same period of illness. Although at the time of the illness behaviour is often grossly disturbed, full recovery is usually seen within a few weeks.

2 Depressive type. Here both schizophrenic and depressive symptoms coexist in the same period of illness. Although the presentation and course of the disease is less florid than that of the manic type, the prognosis is poorer, with patients often being left with persistent symptoms.

3 Mixed type. Here the schizophrenic symptoms coexist with symptoms of mixed bipolar disorder.

These conditions have similarities in symptoms and progression in many cases and we can consider the physiological aspects of psychosis as a whole in the next part of this chapter. Our main focus will be on schizophrenia as it is the predominant condition you will see in clinical practice.

The physiology of psychosis

Many theories have been put forward to try to explain the altered physiology that occurs in psychotic conditions such as schizophrenia; however, the exact physiology remains poorly understood. The most popular and best investigated hypotheses are around the effects and actions of the monoamines dopamine and glutamate in the brain. It is acknowledged that genetic and environmental factors can be contributory to the onset and severity of symptoms. There have also been links with drug and substance use and misuse.

The dopamine hypothesis of schizophrenia

The hypothesis that the monoamine and neurotransmitter dopamine was involved in schizophrenia was first postulated by Carlsson and Lindqvist in 1963. This neurotransmitter and the condition itself have been investigated over the years and a firm link established. Many of the medications we use in psychosis today have their actions on the dopaminergic systems within the brain and central nervous system and this action is responsible for amelioration of the symptoms of the condition but also for many of the side-effects associated with the drugs we use.

In essence the theory tells us that although it cannot explain all of the symptoms and manifestations of the psychotic disorders it plays a large and significant part in the physiological changes that occur and in the treatment used.

The condition is due to an over-activity of the dopaminergic neurones in the brain leading to increased activity or hyperactivity of the system and an abundance of dopamine stimulation of receptors. The receptors involved are located in all parts of the brain but we can look at some of the localized areas affected and relate them to symptoms that occur. Figure 8.1 shows these regions of the brain.

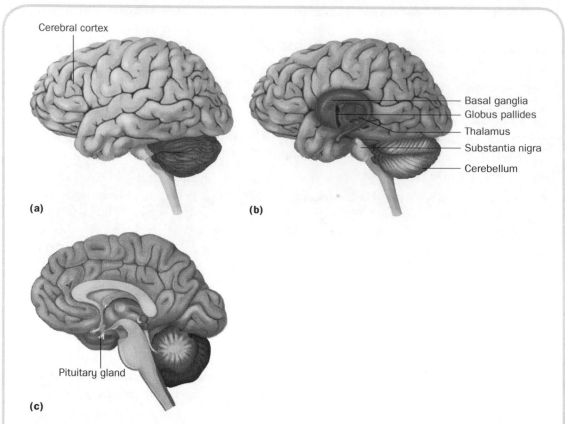

Figure 8.1   Dopamine regions of the brain. (a) The cortex and the limbic system are part of the mesolimbic pathway and are linked to some of the psychological effects seen in psychosis. (b) The basal ganglia and the striatum form part of the nigrostriatal pathway and are linked to movement. (c) The pituitary gland is part of the tuberoinfundibular pathway and is linked to endocrine effects.

The antipsychotic actions and extra-pyramidal side-effects of neuroleptic drugs are strongly correlated with their ability to block central dopaminergic transmission giving credence to the theory. It has also been seen that drugs that can increase dopamine activity in the brain give rise to positive symptoms of schizophrenia.

There are many dopamine receptor types:

- most typical antipsychotics act at D_2 receptors;
- most atypical antipsychotics act at D_1 and D_4 receptors.

The glutamate hypothesis of schizophrenia

Glutamate is also a neurotransmitter within the brain and central nervous system. It has its actions at a receptor called the N-methyl-D-aspartate receptor. Drugs and chemicals that can act at these receptors for glutamate in the brain can give rise to the negative symptoms of schizophrenia. There is a reduction in the activity of glutamate at the receptors and this reduced activity has been linked to frontal lobe function and some of the functions of the hippocampus. It is construed not to be the root cause but more of a mediating or contributory factor. Indeed, as some of the effect of glutamatergic transmission is linked to dopamine systems it may be the interaction between the two systems that is important. Recreational drugs like ketamine and phencyclidine (PCP or angel dust) have been seen to produce psychological states similar to that seen in schizophrenia.

Genetic factors – twin studies

Twin studies have been used to study the effect of genetics on the development of schizophrenia. It

Table 8.1 Chance of developing schizophrenia

Relative with schizophrenia	Chance of developing schizophrenia
None	1 in 100 (normal population risk)
1 parent	1 in 10
1 non-identical twin	1 in 8
1 identical twin	1 in 2

Adapted from The Royal College of Psychiatrists (2015, http://www.rcpsych.ac.uk/mental healthinfoforall/problems/schizophrenia/ schizophrenia.aspx)

was seen that schizophrenia and psychosis could 'run' in families but this does not prove a genetic link. Studies looking at twins (fraternal and identical) showed that there is a higher incidence of schizophrenia in the identical twin group showing a genetic or heritable link. Adoption studies have also been used to look at identical twins who may have been separated at birth where one or both are adopted away from the biological parents. These show that identical twins were at elevated risk of both developing schizophrenia even if reared apart, again suggesting a link. This is highly suggestive that there is some biological predisposition to the condition. The Royal College of Psychiatrists suggest that relationship links and the chance of developing schizophrenia are as shown in Table 8.1.

Environmental factors

Environmental factors such as stressors and influences in the normal development of a person can play a part in the development and severity of psychotic disorders such as schizophrenia. These influences can happen during pregnancy, in the early years or in adolescence. It is thought that most schizophrenia can be attributed to a complex interplay of biological, psychological and social factors. One factor from the environment that has been postulated is the response to stress. Stress causes the release of cortisol in the body. This hormone has many functions but too much of it over too long a time can trigger changes in brain chemistry that may in turn predispose to psychosis.

Cannabis use

More recently some researchers and psychiatrists have looked at the correlation between cannabis use and mental health. There is a growing body of evidence that suggests that regular use of the drug can as much as double your normal lifetime risk of developing schizophrenia (the normal lifetime risk is 1 in 100). But it has also been suggested that, rather than cannabis being a trigger for psychosis, perhaps it is that sufferers from schizophrenia are twice as likely to use cannabis?

It does seem from the research that the earlier in their life someone starts to regularly use cannabis, the more likely they are to go on to have a schizophrenic episode but we also know that not every early-life cannabis user will develop the condition.

Stress vulnerability

The stress-vulnerability model relating to psychosis (Zubin & Spring 1977) is often discussed when identification and management of relapse is necessary in the patient with a diagnosis of psychotic disorder. It is based on the premise that the person has an intrinsic ability to deal with stress and to respond but also that this ability can be shaped and determined by other factors and is not uniform. It also proposes that vulnerability can be enhanced when stressful situations occur leading to a relapse in the patient's condition as the stress itself has a direct effect on the brain. This is not isolated to psychosis as a mental health disorder and can be seen in other conditions but a common feature is thought to be present in the underlying mechanisms that occur when stress affects the brain and the chemicals therein. Stress and stressful situations should be factored into mental health assessment in relapse.

Interventions in managing psychosis

Let us now go on to consider the interventions commonly used in the management of psychosis before we approach the pharmacology of the commonly used medicines.

Management of psychosis, schizophrenia and related disorders

The following guidance is based on NICE guidance CG178 published in February 2014 and is for the management of patients over the age of 18 or with an onset of symptoms before the age of 60. Firstly, it is important to recognize the disruption to peoples' lives and the associated social stigma associated with the diagnosis of schizophrenia. There is a greatly increased risk of suicide in the early stages of the disease. In recognition of this it is important to offer as much support as you can to the patient and the carers.

It is recognized that prevention is better than cure and patients felt to be at risk of developing a psychotic illness should be offered individual CBT and possible family intervention to lessen the risk of developing the condition. Where appropriate the offer of interventions used for depression or anxiety disorders might also be of use.

Early intervention in the acute illness is important, but intervention should be offered to all presenting for the first time regardless of their age or the duration of illness. An assessment should be made for potential PTSD. People presenting for the first time with a psychotic illness are likely to have experienced traumatic events relating to the onset of the condition in the period prior to presentation. If this is the case follow the guidance with regard to the treatment of PTSD as well as treating the psychotic episode.

A choice of medication should be reached with the involvement of the service user. This should include a discussion of the benefits and side-effects of the drugs. This includes weight gain and the potential of diabetes, extra-pyramidal effects, the potential effect on cardiac risk, hormonal effects such as raised prolactin levels, and subjective effects such as the feelings of blunting of emotions. In the initial stages regular combination antipsychotic therapies should be avoided.

Remember that talking therapies and supportive measures should still be offered where appropriate in the management of the acute stages of the disease. Family interventions may also be useful as this may lessen the disruptive impact an acute episode may have on the service user, the carers and the family.

The physical wellbeing of a patient who has or has had a psychotic illness should be monitored closely and an annual health check should be conducted by the patient's GP once they have been handed back into the care of the community services.

The use of clozapine should be considered in patients with schizophrenia who have not responded to adequate treatment with at least two different antipsychotic medications at an adequate therapeutic dose, one of which should be a non-clozapine second-generation antipsychotic medication.

Before starting antipsychotic medication it is important to record the following baseline measurements:

1. weight;

2. waist circumference;

3. pulse and blood pleasure;

4. fasting blood glucose, haemoglobin A_{1c} (HbA$_{1c}$), lipid profile and prolactin level;

5. an assessment of movement disorders;

6. an assessment of nutritional status.

Consider offering an electrocardiogram (ECG) if it is suggested by the drug's summary of product characteristics, or if the physical examination or patient history is suggestive of increased cardiac risk, or if the patient is being admitted as an inpatient.

Once drug treatment is started it should be treated as a therapeutic trial with the following conditions.

1. Initially use a dose at the lower end of the recommended therapeutic range.

2. Justify and record reasons for using a dose outwith those recommended in the BNF.

3. Record the rationale for continuing, stopping or changing medication.

4. Discuss and record the side-effects the patient is willing to tolerate.

5   Record the indications, risks and expected benefits of treatment including timescales.

6   Carry out the medication trial at the optimal dose for four to six weeks.

Monitor and record the following parameters.

1   Response to treatment, changes in symptoms and behaviour.

2   The side-effects of treatment and their impact on functioning.

3   Any emerging movement disorders.

4   Weight. Initial measurement of weight should be weekly for the first 6 weeks, then at 12 weeks then annually.

5   Waist circumference annually.

6   Pulse and blood pressure at 12 weeks and then annually.

7   Bloods (as above) at 12 weeks and then annually.

8   Adherence to treatment.

9   Overall physical health.

Remember to discuss drug and alcohol use and address any issues arising from this. Rapid neuroleptization, where a loading dose of antipsychotic medication is used, is no longer regarded as appropriate.

The use of depot/long-acting injectable antipsychotic medication may be considered. It may be the patient's preference. It may be needed to prevent covert non-adherence.

In patients who do not respond to treatment consider reviewing the diagnosis in light of non-response to medication. Ensure that there

When commencing this type of treatment:

1   Take into account the patient's preference and attitude towards the route of administration and the organizational considerations that go with this (where and when the injections are to be given).

2   Take into account the same criteria outlined for the choice and commencement of oral antipsychotic medication.

3   Initially use a small test dose as outlined in the BNF.

has been compliance with treatment by investigating medication-taking behaviour as part of medicines management or a medication review. It would then be prudent to review the psychological treatments that have been offered and ensure that they comply with the guidance for management of schizophrenia and related disorders. It is also highly appropriate for you to consider the presence of any confounding or comorbid conditions such as drug or alcohol misuse that may not have been previously detected.

We will now go on to have a look at the pharmacological mechanisms of action of some of the most commonly used antipsychotic medication that you will see in your nursing practice.

Pharmacology of antipsychotic medication

Antipsychotic medication can be described as falling into two main categories of drug: The typical and atypical antipsychotics. We will look at each category in turn.

The typical antipsychotics

These are the older generation (or first generation) of antipsychotic medication and many have been around for a very long time. Some of them are still in regular clinical use but others have been used less and less over the years with the development of the newer atypical antipsychotics and the fact that the typical group are associated with many more side-effects.

The main drug names that you will see in this category are listed below.

- Chlorpromazine and thioridazine are phenothiazine drugs that produce moderate to strong sedation. They act non-specifically at dopamine, muscarinic, 5-hydroxytryptamine and adrenoceptors.

- Haloperidol and flupentixol have similar effects and have a lower sedative effect than the classical phenothiazines. They act at dopamine, 5-hydroxytryptamine, muscarinic and adrenoceptors.
- Fluphenazine, prochlorperazine and trifluoperazine are generally categorized by fewer sedative and antimuscarinic effects but have more pronounced extra-pyramidal effects. They have the majority of their effects through dopamine blockade but there are some adrenergic effects.
- Sulpiride is a dopamine and 5-hydroxytryptamine blocker and is effective in the treatment of schizophrenia.

Many of these drugs have been used since the 1950s and we are quite familiar with them and their actions. Their main mechanism of action is blockade of the dopamine D_2 receptor. This means that although dopamine is still present and being released into the synapse it cannot have its full effect at the receptors because they are blocked by the presence of the drug molecule. As considered in the section on physiology, dopamine activity is heavily implicated in schizophrenia and this would explain why these drugs have been so effective in reducing the symptoms of psychosis.

Dopamine D_2 receptors are located in many areas of the brain and their blockade can also cause significant side-effects. Other dopamine receptors are also involved (see Figure 8.2). We can relate some of the effects and side-effects to the areas of the brain we looked at earlier.

Dopamine receptors:

- D_1 found in the frontal cortex;
- D_2 and D_4 are widespread;
- D_3 linked to limbic system;
- D_5 has no link to schizophrenia.

The mesolimbic pathway

The blockade of dopamine D_2 receptors here is responsible for much of the antipsychotic mechanism of the drug but is also responsible for side-effects such as sedation and impaired performance. This can be prolonged and intolerable to patients and they complain of feeling 'fuzzy' or 'foggy' relating to clouding of their thought processes. It is one of the reasons patients are less tolerant of these types of medication.

The nigrostriatal pathway

When we have D_2 receptor blockade in this region we see side-effects related to movement. These typically manifest as dystonia or dyskinesia and some are said to be 'Parkinson like' in their form. A severe side-effect that comes with long-term use of these medications is the irreversible effect of tardive dyskinesia. We will look at these so called extra-pyramidal side-effects later.

The tuberoinfudibular pathway

This area has endocrine effects and when we block D_2 receptors here we see effects on the neuro-endocrine system. Typical side-effects are amenorrhoea, galactorrhoea, hyperprolactinaemia, gynaecomastia and infertility. These symptoms are usually transient and will reverse on discontinuation of the drug.

We also see a high incidence of cholinergic side-effects with these drugs as they have actions on other transmitter systems as well as their main action at dopamine D_2. These effects include dry mouth, blurred vision, constipation, urinary retention and ejaculatory failure. We can also see other effects on adrenergic systems such as low blood pressure and heart beat irregularities. And there are other miscellaneous symptoms that have been

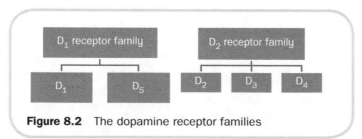

Figure 8.2 The dopamine receptor families

frequently reported such as sensitivity to heat and sunlight, jaundice, pigmentation of the retina and the serious neuroleptic malignant syndrome.

However, you can see that such side-effects, all of which occur with medium to high frequency, can be quite debilitating, inconvenient or intolerable to the patient. Some are life affecting. It is for this reason that many patients that you will come across in your current practice are now treated with and managed on the newer atypical antipsychotics.

The atypical antipsychotics

These are the newer generation (or second generation) of antipsychotic medication.

- Amisulpride has its actions primarily at dopamine D_2 and D_3 receptors with a high affinity for both. There is also some activity at 5-hydroxytryptamine receptors.
- Clozapine is a dibenzodiazepine neuroleptic and exerts its effect via dopamine receptors and 5-hydroxytryptamine receptors with some adrenergic effect seen also. It is associated with some serious potential side-effects. It is effective in depression and anxiety and the negative symptoms seen in schizophrenia.
- Olanzapine has a high affinity for 5-hydroxytryptamine receptors but also exerts effects at dopamine D_1, D_2 and D_4 as well as muscarinic receptors. It is associated with side-effects.
- Quetiapine is effective against positive symptoms and has activity mainly at dopamine D_1 receptors and 5-hydroxytryptamine receptors with some adrenergic and muscarinic effects. It is associated with many side-effects.
- Risperidone has a higher affinity for 5-hydroxytryptamine than dopamine and has a lower incidence of extra-pyramidal side-effects than other neuroleptics.
- Aripiprazole has activity at dopamine D_2 and 5-hydroxytryptamine receptors. It is associated with fewer side-effects than many other antipsychotics.

Side-effects of atypical antipsychotics

Like their typical counterparts the atypical antipsychotics do have side-effects and, although there are fewer than for the typical ones, some of them are still serious and undesirable. Amisulpride is associated with a very common incidence of extra-pyramidal side-effects. Clozapine, as you can see from above, is linked to some serious side-effects and it is because of these that careful initiation and monitoring of treatment should take place. Some of the side-effects are potentially fatal so it is important that signs of these are looked for in a patient receiving clozapine treatment. These include agranulocytosis (an acute and severe reduction in the number of white blood cells) and cardiac toxicity leading to myocarditis. Other side-effects can be viewed as serious but less life threatening. Weight gain is common and in some this causes a diabetes-like state. The central nervous system is affected and drowsiness and vertigo are common; seizures are possible but rarer. These side-effects are usually transient and resolve on stopping the drug.

Olanzapine has a number of side-effects you need to be aware of. Its principle undesired effect is weight gain and this can be quite rapid and significant in some cases. It increases appetite, which compounds the problem. It is also associated with some extra-pyramidal effects and can cause derangement of blood levels of glucose and lipids. Monitoring is advised.

Quetiapine has numerous side-effects but many common side-effects are through muscarinic actions and include dry mouth. There is a fairly common incidence of changes to blood pressure; this can be raised or lowered and regular blood pressure monitoring is advised. Serious, but thankfully rare, effects include cardiac events and blood dyscrasias. Aripiprazole is associated with side-effects of anxiety and some hypersalivation. Tolerability is good.

Extra-pyramidal side-effects

We have mentioned these in association with many of the antipsychotic drugs and it is worth explaining this concept a little more fully. Extrapyramidal side-effects are effects induced by certain medications, the antipsychotics being the commonest, and they produce disorder of movement. They are usually assessed for severity by the use of rating scales. They include the following categories:

- dystonia – muscular spasms;
- akathisia – motor restlessness;
- Parkinson-like effects – rigidity and tremor;
- tardive dyskinesia – facial involuntary movements in long-term and chronic use.

It is important that you gain a working familiarity with these medications used in practice. You should be able to use the BNF to look up the medicines and to ascertain any effects and side-effects your patients may experience. You should also be able to use Appendix One of the BNF to check for interactions that these medications may have with other medications your patient may be taking at the same time.

Key learning points

Psychosis

▶ Schizophrenia is the commonest form of psychotic disorder.

Physiology and pharmacology

▶ The aetiology and pathophysiology of schizophrenia has not been completely explained.
▶ Dopamine and glutamate are two monoamine transmitters implicated in psychotic disorder.
▶ Environmental and genetic factors can contribute to the onset and severity of symptoms of psychosis.
▶ The choice of antipsychotic medication should be made following guidelines and jointly between the prescriber and the patient.
▶ Monitoring of patients on antipsychotic medication is necessary not just for effect but to assess incidence and severity of side-effects.

Drug calculations

1 Your patient is prescribed haloperidol 3mg tablets three times per day. You have 1.5mg tablets.

How many tablets per dose?

How many tablets per day?

How many tablets for a 28-day supply?

2 Your patient requires aripiprazole 15mg daily. You have 5mg tablets.

How many tablets per day?

How many tablets for a 28-day supply?

3 Your patient requires olanzapine 10mg daily. You have 2.5mg tablets.

How many tablets per day?

How many tablets for a 28-day supply? →

4 Your patient is prescribed clozapine 300mg in two divided doses per day. You have 25mg tablets.

How many tablets per dose?

How many tablets per day?

How many tablets for a 28-day supply?

5 Your patient requires sulpiride 400mg twice daily. You have 40mg per ml solution.

How many ml per dose?

How many ml per day?

How many ml for a 28-day supply?

6 Your patient is prescribed amisulpride 200mg twice daily. You have 50mg tablets.

How many tablets per day?

How many tablets for a 28-day supply?

7 Your patient requires quetiapine 25mg twice daily on day one, 50mg twice daily on day two, 100mg twice daily on day 3 and then 150mg twice daily for the rest of the prescription. You have 25mg tablets.

How many tablets for day one?

How many tablets for day two?

How many tablets for day three?

How many tablets for day four and all subsequent days?

How many tablets to be supplied in total for 28-days?

8 Your patient requires risperidone 12.5mg by deep IM injection. You have 25mg per ml powder for reconstitution in solution.

How many ml will you give?

9 Your patient is prescribed paliperidone 9mg daily. You have 3mg tablets.

How many tablets per day?

How many tablets for a 28-day supply?

10 Your patient is prescribed lurasidone 148mg daily. You have 37mg tablets.

How many tablets per dose?

How many tablets for a 28-day supply?

Multiple choice questions

Try answering these multiple choice questions to test what you have learned from reading this chapter. You can check your answers on page 153.

1 Antipsychotic medication can be classed as

   a) Simple and complex
   b) Typical and atypical
   c) Sedating and non-sedating
   d) Therapeutic and prophylactic

2 What class does the drug haloperidol belong to?

   a) Atypical
   b) Simple
   c) Complex
   d) Typical

3 What class does the drug aripiprazole belong to?

   a) Atypical
   b) Simple
   c) Complex
   d) Typical

4 Which monoamine is most associated with schizophrenia?

   a) 5-hydroxytryptamine
   b) Noradrenaline
   c) Adrenaline
   d) Dopamine

5 Overdose of antipsychotic medication can cause side-effects similar to symptoms of

   a) Epilepsy
   b) Parkinson's disease
   c) Diabetes
   d) Anxiety

6 What is the most common form of psychosis?

   a) Paranoid schizophrenia
   b) Schizoaffective disorder
   c) Hebephrenic schizophrenia
   d) Catatonic schizophrenia

$\longrightarrow$

7 What is the number of the NICE guideline relating to the management of schizophrenia?

   a) CG178
   b) CG113
   c) CG90
   d) CG91

8 Olanzapine acts at what kind of receptors?

   a) Dopamine
   b) Serotonin
   c) Muscarinic
   d) All of the above

9 Clozapine is useful in schizophrenia with

   a) Predominantly positive symptoms
   b) Predominantly negative symptoms
   c) A mix of negative and positive symptoms
   d) Depression also present

10 The choice of antipsychotic medication should be

   a) Made by the doctor
   b) Made by the patient
   c) Made using guidelines
   d) All of the above

Case study

Benita White is a 24-year-old student of mixed Afro-Caribbean descent. She has a diagnosis of paranoid schizophrenia and her current medication is olanzapine. She has recently started at university and is working hard at her coursework and socializing with new friends. She is taking her medication but admits she has not been doing so regularly or always at the correct dose. She has been hearing voices telling her that her classmates are out to get her. She wants new drugs to make the voices stop.

■ Outline the initial approach you as a nurse could take in her management and what you might suggest for Benita.

Recommended websites

British National Formulary (BNF): www.bnf.org
EMC medicines compendium: www.medicines.org.uk
www.rethink.org

Recommended further reading

Carlsson, A. and Lindqvist, M. (1963) Effect of chlorpromazine or haloperidol on the formation of 3-methoxytyramine and normetanephrine in mouse brain. *Acta Pharmacologica* 20: 140–144.

National Institute for Health and Care Excellence (NICE) (2014) *Psychosis and Schizophrenia in Adults: Prevention and Management. CG178.* Available at: https://www.nice.org.uk/guidance/cg178 (accessed 23 February 2016).

Royal College of Psychiatrists (2015) *Schizophrenia.* London: Royal College of Psychiatrists. Available at: http://www.rcpsych.ac.uk/mentalhealthinfoforall/problems/schizophrenia/schizophrenia.aspx (accessed 22 February 2016).

World Health Organization (WHO) (2016) *International Statistical Classification of Diseases and Related Health Problems 10th Revision (ICD-10) – WHO Version for 2016.* Available at: http://apps.who.int/classifications/icd10/browse/2016/en (accessed 19 February 2016).

Zubin, J. and Spring, B. (1977) Vulnerability: a new view of schizophrenia. *Journal of Abnormal Psychology* 86: 103–126.

Dementia and disorders in the older adult

9

Chapter contents

Learning objectives

After reading this chapter you will have gained knowledge around:

- The group of conditions categorized as dementias.
- The physiology and pharmacology around dementia.
- The pharmacodynamic actions of drugs used in dementia.

Introduction

Dementia is a disease of the brain in which there is disruption of the higher cortical functions such as memory, language, learning ability, comprehension and judgement. This is usually chronic and progressive in nature. Consciousness is not diminished. Usually there is also a deterioration in emotional control and motivation that can lead to a deterioration in social functioning. This may accompany the deterioration in cognitive function or may pre-date it. Many of these symptoms are also seen with other mental health issues and also with some physical illnesses and care should be taken to exclude conditions such as depression or hypothyroid disease before a diagnosis of dementia is made.

The diagnosis of dementia is made initially on evidence of a decline in memory and cognitive functioning significant enough to impair the ability to undertake the tasks of daily living. Typically memory impairment shows as an increasing inability to process, store and retrieve new information. Older memories, such as those of childhood, may be spared in the early stages, but may well be lost as the disease progresses. There is also a disruption in cognition and reasoning that can interfere with the flow of ideas. In essence we see:

- cognitive changes;
- physical changes;
- emotional changes;
- behavioural changes.

There are many forms of dementia that we shall outline here; however, the predominant form is Alzheimer's disease and this fact will determine much of the focus of this chapter.

The classifications of dementia

Alzheimer's disease

This is a degenerative cerebral disease where there is no recognized underlying cause. There are, however, recognized neuropathological and neurochemical features. There is typically an insidious onset over a period of years. This may be rapid over a couple of years or may be more prolonged. The onset of the disease may be in the third

or fourth decade of life but is typically later. The incidence of the disease increases with age and it seems to be more common in patients with Down's syndrome. The progress of the disease tends to be slower in those who develop it later in life.

Diagnosis is made on the basis of the clinical findings uncovered by the doctor during consultation and examination. This means that it is made on the basis of the criteria laid out above when there is an insidious onset of symptoms associated with a slow deterioration. The exact onset of symptoms may be difficult to place due to the insidious nature of the illness. Remember that it is necessary to exclude other conditions that might mimic the symptoms of dementia. For diagnostic purposes, Alzheimer's disease has been subdivided into two categories: first, early onset, beginning before the age of 65 years, and second, late onset where the onset of symptoms happens after the age of 65 years. There appears to be a difference in the progression of the disease with early-onset Alzheimer's patients suffering a more rapid progression of the disease with features of temporal and parietal lobe damage such as dysphasia and dyspraxia. Patients with the later onset variant tend to show a slower progression with a more global deterioration of higher cortical function. People with Alzheimer's disease live an average of 8 years, but some people may survive up to 20 years.

Alzheimer's disease itself can be further sub-classified:

- mild;
- moderate;
- severe.

Vascular dementia/multi-infarct dementia

Here there is disruption in the blood supply to areas of the brain producing focal neuron loss. This is associated with arteriopathy and hypertension. It is typically associated with recurrent transient ischaemic attacks, but is also seen with recurrent cerebrovascular accidents and, on occasions, with one-off major strokes. There is a stepwise progression of the disease with every infarct resulting in a further deterioration in function. Because of the focal nature of the condition loss of cognitive function may be patchy. For example, there may be memory loss and intellectual impairment without impairment of insight.

Dementia with Lewy bodies

This form of dementia shares much of its cognitive decline features with Alzheimer's disease; however, in many cases symptoms of Parkinson's disease are also seen. It is thought to account for a not insignificant 10 to 15 per cent of all diagnosed dementias (Acampa & Navti 2014). The Lewy body is a protein deposit seen on nerve cells. This is associated with decreased levels of neurotransmitters such as acetylcholine and dopamine. As the disease progresses, nerve cell death is a feature.

Pick's disease

This is a progressive form of dementia usually presenting between the ages of 50 and 60 years. It typically has a slow progression and is characterized by impairment of intellect, memory and language functions. It may also be associated with extra-pyramidal symptoms. The neuropathology is that of a selective atrophy of the frontal and temporal lobes, which is more than would be expected in the normal aging process. Also there is an absence of the plaques and tangles associated with Alzheimer's disease. However, like Alzheimer's disease, early onset is associated with a more rapid progression of the illness.

Other causes

Dementia is also seen as a feature of other degenerative brain diseases. These include Creutzfeldt–Jakob disease, Huntington's disease, Parkinson's disease and human immunodeficiency virus (HIV) disease – although this is not an exclusive list.

For further reading look at ICD-10 classification (WHO 2016), sections F00 to F03.

The physiology of dementia

Alzheimer's disease

The neuropathological features of the disease include a reduction in the population of neurons in the hippocampus, the substantia innominate, the locus coeruleus and the temporo-parietal and frontal cortices. Neurofibrillary tangles and plaques, some of which may contain amyloid, are also seen. The neurochemical changes involve acetylcholine and include a reduction in the enzyme choline acetyltransferase and also in acetylcholine itself. Other neurotransmitters and neuromodulating chemicals may also be reduced. These features are also progressive, but the rate of progression of the neuropathological and neurochemical features may not correlate to the progression of the symptoms displayed by the patient.

The cortex area of the brain appears shrivelled, which can cause damage to the areas principally concerned with thinking, planning and remembering. There is shrinkage in other key brain regions and it is often severe in the hippocampus, an area you will remember from Chapter 5 that plays a key role in the formation of new memories.

There is usually significant disruption to cholinergic transmission, and this can be at the level of the neurotransmitter acetylcholine and at the level of the receptors it acts upon.

It is also known that microscopy can identify the effects of Alzheimer's disease when post-mortem brain tissue is examined and the following defining features can be seen.

- Tissue affected by Alzheimer's disease has fewer nerve cells and synapses than healthy areas of the brain.
- Plaques, aggregations of protein fragments, are observed between nerve cells.
- Dead and dying nerve cells are present and these contain tangles made up of twisted strands of protein.

These plaques and tangles tend to spread throughout the brain in a systematic and predictable pattern as the disease progresses.

Now that we have outlined the classification and physiology of the dementias we will explore the range of interventions available in these conditions.

Interventions in managing dementia

Interventions can only be considered after a firm diagnosis has been made. A diagnosis of dementia can only be made after the patient has undergone a physical examination as well as a cognitive and mental state examination. This will include haematological and biochemical studies. An assessment of the patient's drug history is also essential. It has to be remembered that there are a number of conditions that can mimic the symptoms of dementia and these treatable conditions have to be excluded before a diagnosis of dementia can be made. It should also be remembered that there are a number of disease processes that have dementia as part of the recognized pathology of the condition and this may be useful in determining the type of dementia and the future management of the condition.

To help with the diagnosis of dementia, once other conditions have been excluded, there are a number of tests available. You should familiarize yourself with the tests available and particularly with those used in your local area. These may include The Mini-Mental State Examination (or MMSE), the 6-item Cognitive Impairment Test (or 6-CIT), the General Practitioner's Assessment of Cognition test (or GPCOG) and the Seven Minute Screen. When using any test for the assessment of cognition it is important to take into account other issues that may affect the patient's level of functioning such as educational attainment, language, previous psychiatric illness or concomitant physical disease, all of which may have an adverse effect on the patient's performance.

The aim of managing dementia patients is to maintain their independence for as long as possible. In attempting to do this there are a number of factors that have been recognized as important. It is important to maintain stability within the home setting. Familiar surroundings and the use of the same carers helps to maintain this. When moves or changes do occur it is important to minimize the number of changes, for example moving a patient through several care homes over a short period of time will have a greater adverse effect on their functioning than a single move. An assessment by an appropriately trained professional, preferably an occupational therapist, of the patient's ability to perform the activities of daily living and the use of appropriate aids or alterations to the home environment, if needed, will help maintain function and dig-

nity, as will a formal assessment of continence and the use of appropriate continence aids. Due to the progressive nature of the condition there also has to be a degree of flexibility in the approach that allows it to adapt to fluctuations in the patient's abilities. It is important to state that inclusion of any family members in the planning and delivery of this care is essential as they may form the primary carers for the patient. Having said that it is also important to maintain confidentiality where appropriate and to respect the patient's own wishes, and assessment of capacity should be made where appropriate (refer to Chapter 2 for more on legal and ethical issues related to mental capacity).

Medication can be prescribed as long as benefits are deemed to be achievable. In patients with mild to moderate Alzheimer's disease acetylcholinesterase inhibitors, such as donepezil, galantamine and rivastigmine, can be used. In the patient with moderate to severe Alzheimer's disease or in patients who have not been able to tolerate acetylcholinesterase inhibitors, or in those where these drugs are contraindicated, memantine may be used. There have been some benefits seen with this drug, which is a glutamate receptor antagonist.

Treatment should only be initiated after an assessment by a specialist in this area. Treatment then should only be continued if it is seen to be beneficial with an improvement seen in global cognitive functioning or a lessening of any behavioural problems. To allow this to be properly assessed, regular review using the appropriate assessment tools should be undertaken.

In the management of the non-Alzheimer's type dementias the aim is predominantly supportive. Where appropriate any risk factors that might be present for progression of the disease should be addressed. These risk factors would include the need for optimal management of the cardiovascular risks in patients who have multi-infarct dementia, and also the need to use antiviral drugs to limit the progress of the disease in patients who also have HIV. There are some forms of dementia for which there is no effective way to limit the progression of the disease and in these cases supportive measures may be all that is available to help these patients. Symptom control is also important. For example, patients with Huntington's disease will be prone to depression as they attempt to come to terms with the diagnosis and this will in turn affect cognitive function. Treating this depression may lead to an improvement in function.

Non-pharmacological interventions to improve sleep hygiene and routine are often used. These can include:

- routine times for things such as meals and retiring to bed;
- regular exercise, where appropriate;
- avoidance of stimulants such as alcohol, caffeine and nicotine especially near bedtime;
- treat any pain that may be being experienced;
- if an acetylcholinesterase inhibitor medication is prescribed, avoid administration of this immediately prior to the patient going to bed;
- make sure the bedroom temperature is comfortable and any security objects are present (teddy bear, comforter);
- if the person awakens, discourage staying in bed while awake; use the bed only for sleep and discourage watching television during periods of wakefulness or in bed;
- discourage daytime naps.

Further information on all of this can be found in NICE guidelines CG16 (2015) and CG42 (2006).

Pharmacology of medication used in dementia

Let us look in more detail at the medications mentioned above and consider the aspects of the management of dementia they address.

Medication for memory loss

Cholinesterase inhibitors such as donepezil, galantamine and rivastigmine have been used with varying degrees of success. These drugs are predominantly prescribed in mild to moderate Alzheimer's disease and can slow the cognitive decline thereby slowing the progression of the condition. Treatment must be initiated and supervized by an experienced clinician in this area of psychiatric practice. Assessment of effect should be made after three months of treatment and the medications discontinued if the patient is not seen to be responding.

Donepezil is the only cholinesterase inhibitor approved to treat all stages of Alzheimer's disease, including moderate to severe. It is a reversible inhibitor of acetylcholinesterase. This means that it reduces the enzyme responsible for the breakdown of the neurotransmitter acetylcholine and prolongs its presence in the synapse and its action at receptors. This is thought to be its primary mechanism of action in slowing cognitive decline.

Galantamine is also a reversible inhibitor of acetylcholinesterase and in addition it has agonist activity at nicotinic receptors. It is licensed for use in mild to moderate disease and its actions are predominantly related to its activity as an acetylcholinesterase inhibitor.

Rivastigmine is also a reversible inhibitor of acetylcholinesterase but its action is non-competitive in nature. This means it does not have to bind to acetylcholine to have its effect on the enzyme that is responsible for its breakdown. Again it is used in mild to moderate disease.

Memantine is another drug that can be prescribed to improve function or lessen cognitive decline. It does not inhibit acetylcholinesterase but has its effects at glutamate receptors. It can be used alone or in conjunction with other medications. There is some evidence that individuals with moderate to severe Alzheimer's disease who are taking a cholinesterase inhibitor might benefit by also taking memantine.

Like any medications these drugs can cause side-effects, including headache, constipation, confusion and dizziness, so careful monitoring is required and medicines optimization is important (Acampa and Navti 2014).

Further information on the prescribing of these medications can be found in the NICE technical appraisal document TA217 (NICE 2011).

Treatment of behavioural changes

In the early stages of the disease, people may experience or have perceived changes to their behaviour and personality including:

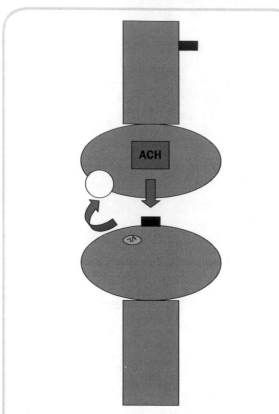

Figure 9.1   Diagram showing acetylcholinesterase release and actions of drugs on the system. Key: neurons are in dark grey; arrow dictates route of release and reuptake of acetylcholine (ACH); black boxes are receptors; clear circle is the reuptake system; the light grey oval is acetylcholinesterase.

- irritability and/or agitation;
- anxiety;
- depression.

In the later stages of the disease, other symptoms may be encountered including:

- anger;
- agitation;
- aggression;
- general emotional distress;
- physical or verbal outbursts;
- restlessness, pacing, shredding paper or tissues;
- hallucinations and/or delusions.

In extreme, severe or prevailing cases then pharmacological management of these symptoms is appropriate. Medication used tends to fall into the following categories:

- anxiolytics (refer to Chapter 6);
- antidepressants (refer to Chapter 7);
- antipsychotics (refer to Chapter 8).

Treatment of sleep disturbance

Sleep disturbance can be a significant issue, and pharmacological help with sleep is often appropriate and occurs in cases where non-pharmacological interventions have been less than successful and/or the sleep changes are accompanied by disruptive or unsafe night-time behaviours and so pharmacological intervention is necessary. This is, however, not without attendant risk, and many things have to be considered before prescribing of a hypnotic drug occurs.

Risks include falls and fractures, confusion or agitation and at times a reduction in the normal activities of daily living. If a hypnotic is used, this should be as a short-term intervention and once a more normal sleep pattern has returned then the medication should be stopped.

Medications that may be used include the following.

- The tricyclic antidepressants, such as nortriptyline and trazodone.
- The benzodiazepines, such as lorazepam and temazepam.
- Z-drug hypnotics such as zolpidem, zopiclone and zaleplon.
- Atypical antipsychotics such as risperidone, olanzapine and quetiapine.
- Typical antipsychotics such as haloperidol.

You should be aware of the increase in cardiovascular risk for the patient when antipsychotics are used. It is important that you gain a working familiarity with these medications used in practice. You should be able to use the BNF to look up the medicines and to ascertain any effects and side-effects your patients may experience. You should also be able to use Appendix One of the BNF to check for interactions that these medications may have with other medications that your patient may be taking at the same time.

Key learning points

Classifications of dementia

▶ The nurse should be aware of the different types of dementia that exist.
▶ Alzheimer's disease is the most prevalent form in UK society.

Physiology and pharmacology

▶ The physiology of dementia is complex with many chemical and structural changes to the brain and central nervous system.
▶ Symptoms and signs are multiple in nature and depend on the progression of the disease as well as the classification of dementia.
▶ Pharmacology in dementia is limited with regard to the slowing of cognitive decline.
▶ Much of the medication given is for symptom management or control.

Drug calculations

1 Your patient requires temazepam 10mg at night. You have 2mg per ml oral solution.

How many ml per dose?

How many ml for a 28-day supply?

2 Your patient requires zolpidem 5mg at night. You have 5mg tablets.

How many tablets per day?

How many tablets for a 14-day supply?

3 Your patient requires galantamine 12mg twice daily. You have 8mg scored tablets.

How many tablets per day?

How many tablets for a 28-day supply?

4 Your patient requires donepezil 10mg daily. You have 1mg per ml solution.

How many ml per dose?

How many ml for a 28-day supply?

5 Your patient requires rivastigmine in a 13.3mg patch over a 24-hour period. How much rivastigmine is released per hour from the patch?

6 Your patient requires memantine 20mg per day. You have a 50ml bottle of 10mg per ml solution.

How long will this bottle last?

7 Your patient requires trazodone 300mg daily. You have 50mg capsules.

How many capsules per day?

How many capsules for a 28-day supply?

8 Your patient requires haloperidol 1mg as required for agitation but can have no more than two doses per day. You have a box of 28 × 500microgram tablets.

If the drug is given at its maximum daily dose how long will this box last?

9 Your patient requires risperidone 250micrograms twice daily. You have 0.5mg scored tablets.

How many tablets per dose?

How many tablets per day?

How many tablets for a 28-day supply?

10 Your patient requires olanzapine 15mg daily. You have 7.5mg tablets.

How many tablets per day?

How many tablets for a 28-day supply?

Multiple choice questions

Try answering these multiple choice questions to test what you have learned from reading this chapter. You can check your answers on page 154.

1 What is the most common form of dementia you will encounter?

a) Alzheimer's disease
b) Lewy body dementia
c) Vascular dementia
d) Pick's disease

2 What are the numbers of the NICE clinical guidelines used in the management of dementia?

a) CGs 15 and 42
b) CGs 16 and 42
c) CGs 15 and 43
d) CGs 16 and 43

3 What features characterize Alzheimer's disease?

a) Lewy bodies
b) Plaques
c) Tangles
d) Plaques and tangles

4 Cholinesterase enzyme acts on which neurotransmitter?

a) Dopamine
b) Serotonin

c) Adrenaline
d) Acetylcholine

5 When can hypnotics for sleep be used?

a) When a patient requests them
b) When a carer requests them
c) If a patient is in pain
d) When non-pharmacological measures have been ineffective

6 What receptor does memantine act on?

a) Cholinergic
b) Nicotinic
c) Serotonergic
d) Glutamate

7 Which cholinesterase inhibitor is licensed for all stages of Alzheimer's disease?

a) Donepezil
b) Galantamine
c) Rivastigmine
d) Memantine

8 Which of the following behaviour changes can be seen in early dementia?

a) Depression
b) Anxiety
c) Agitation
d) All of the above

9 Much of the medication used in dementia care is for

a) Reduction in cognitive decline
b) Symptom management
c) Reversal of the condition
d) Palliation

10 Which of these is a major risk when prescribing hypnotics in dementia?

a) Falls
b) Drowsiness
c) Shock
d) Cognitive relapse

Case study

Mabel Anderson is a 79-year-old lady who suffers from Alzheimer's disease. She lives with her husband who has noticed a steady decline in her memory and cognitive abilities. She meets the criteria in the NICE guidelines for commencing an acetylcholinesterase inhibitor. What points should be considered when she commences the medication?

Recommended websites

Alzheimer's Association (USA): www.alz.org
Alzheimer's Society (UK): https://www.alzheimers.org.uk/
British National Formulary (BNF): www.bnf.org
EMC medicines compendium: www.medicines.org.uk

Recommended further reading

Acampa, B. and Navti, B. (2014) Medicines optimization in the dementias. *Nurse Prescribing* 12(11): 557–563.

National Institute for Health and Care Excellence (NICE) (2006) *Dementia: Supporting People with Dementia and their Carers in Health and Social Care. CG42.* London: NICE. Available at: https://www.nice.org.uk/guidance/cg42 (accessed 23 February 2016).

National Institute for Health and Care Excellence (NICE) (2011) *Donepezil, Galantamine, Rivastigmine and Memantine for the Treatment of Alzheimer's Disease. Technical appraisal: TA217.* London: NICE. Available at: https://www.nice.org.uk/guidance/ta217 (accessed 23 February 2016).

National Institute for Health and Care Excellence (NICE) (2015) *Dementia, Disability and Frailty in Later Life – Mid-Life Approaches to Delay or Prevent Onset. CG16.* London: NICE. Available at: https://www.nice.org.uk/guidance/ng16 (accessed 23 February 2016).

The Crown Office. (2005) *Mental Capacity Act 2005.* Available at: http://www.legislation.gov.uk/ukpga/2005/9/contents (accessed 23 February 2016).

World Health Organization (WHO)(2016) *International Statistical Classification of Diseases and Related Health Problems 10th Revision (ICD-10) – WHO Version for 2016.* Available at: http://apps.who.int/classifications/icd10/browse/2016/en (accessed 19 February 2016).

Bipolar affective disorder

10

Chapter contents

Learning objectives

After reading this chapter you will have gained knowledge around:

- The incidence and manifestations of bipolar affective disorders.
- The physiology and pharmacology around bipolar affective disorders.
- The complexities of treatment in bipolar affective disorders.
- The pharmacodynamic actions of drugs used in bipolar affective disorders.

Introduction

Bipolar affective disorder is the term used to cover disorders of mood where mania is also present as well as depressed mood being a feature. It used to be described as manic depression, which was a term that encompassed the range of mood that could be seen during a typical cycle of the disorder. This term is very much out of favour now and you will find most people refer to it as bipolar disorder or bipolar affective disorder. The range of conditions will be explored in this chapter as will the understood physiology behind it before we go on to examine the medications used in the treatment and management of these serious and sometimes debilitating disorders.

Bipolar affective disorder

There are many categories of condition that come under this classification of mental health disorder and they have many similarities and associated symptoms.

Hypomania

This is not as severe as mania, but shares the same characteristics. There is persistent elevation of mood with increased energy and activity. This is usually accompanied by an increased feeling of wellbeing and physical and mental efficiency. There may also be increased sociability with over-familiarity and increased sexual energy. There is often a decreased need for sleep. It should be noted that irritability, conceit and boorish behaviour may replace the commoner euphoric sociability. Concentration may be impaired so the ability to work or to take part in more complex activities may be impaired. However, this will not stop the pursuit of new interests or activities. There may also be mild overspending. For the diagnosis to be made, several of the features mentioned above should have been present for at least several days. There may be some disruption to work and social activity, but this is not always severe.

Mania without psychotic symptoms

Here the mood is again elevated beyond the individual's circumstances and may vary from joviality to uncontrollable excitement. This is accompanied by increased energy resulting in over-activity, pressure of speech and a decreased need for sleep. Normal social inhibitions are lost, attention cannot be maintained and the individual will be easily distracted. They may have an inflated self-esteem and express grandiose ideas. They may experience sensations in a more vivid manner. There may be reckless spending and the person may pursue extravagant courses of action. They may behave inappropriately, for example becoming amorous at a funeral. On occasions the elated mood may be replaced with irritability and suspicion. The usual age of onset is between 15 and 30, but it may occur at any age. Any episode should last at least seven days and be associated with severe disruption to normal daily functioning.

Mania with psychotic symptoms

This is as above but with the addition of delusional symptoms. These often involve grandiose schemes or religious identities, although it may also include delusions of persecution. Flight of ideas and pressure of speech may predominate and the individual may neglect to eat or drink for prolonged periods of time due to sustained physical activity. You may want to revise this area of Chapter 8.

True bipolar affective disorder

This is seen when there are two or more episodes of disturbance in mood. These may be seen on one occasion as mania or hypomania and another as depression. There may be periods of normality between these disturbances. Manic episodes tend to have a sudden onset and last about four months. The depressive episodes tend to be more prolonged. They may be triggered by stress, but this is not always true. The onset may be at any age. As the disease progresses the periods of remission between episodes tend to shorten and the periods of depression become more dominant. The condition may be associated with psychotic features, although again this is not always the case.

For further information on the definition and diagnostic criteria for these conditions see the ICD-10 (WHO 2016) sections F30.0 to F31.9.

The physiology of bipolar affective disorder

The exact physiological mechanisms that cause bipolar affective and related disorders of mood is still poorly understood. Many theories have been suggested and much research surrounds the condition. However, it seems that the development of these conditions is down to a complex interplay of biological, psychological, social and environmental factors, not dissimilar to other mental health disorders that we have looked at so far.

Genetic links

Evidence shows that if you have someone in your immediate blood family who has bipolar disorder then this increases your likelihood of developing the disorder. This seems to be more to do with genetics than upbringing. The disorder does appear to 'run' in families. Research has not been able to pinpoint any specific genes that could be said to be defective and that cause the disorder but suggests that a number of factors act as triggers.

Biochemical theories

It is widely thought and reported that the main causative factor in the development of bipolar affective disorder and related conditions is due to chemical instabilities or imbalances within the brain itself. This has been investigated with relation to some of the monoamines and neurotransmitters that we have looked at in other chapters dealing with depression and anxiety and in the chapter on anatomy and physiology of the brain. There have been suggestions of involvement of noradrenaline and adrenaline as well as dopamine and serotonin, but no conclusive links have been made with any one monoamine as causative. However, as we will see some drugs used in the management of this set of conditions do have affects on brain chemistry and monoamine systems lending credence to their involvement in the disorder's manifestation.

Social, psychological and environmental influences

There has been much written about stress and its relationship with bipolar affective disorders. Some researchers believe that stress is the cause of the disorder whereas others acknowledge it plays a part but may be seen more as a trigger or contributory factor. It is known that in people with a diagnosed condition stress can trigger a manic or a depressive event or be responsible for the person entering a rapid cycling phase of their disorder (where the person moves rapidly from depressive state to manic state and back again, sometimes continually).

Sometimes the stressors themselves can be seen as triggers. Stressful life events (even supposedly pleasant events can be stressful), such as work or money problems, relationship issues, house moves and weddings, bereavement and physical illness can also be stress provoking and trigger an event.

Interventions in bipolar affective disorder

Let us next consider the range of options available to manage bipolar disorder.

Management of hypomania, mania and bipolar dicorder

There is emphasis on supportive measures and talking therapies that are suggested in the NICE guidance CG185 for the management of this condition (NICE 2014). There is also a strong suggestion that commencing drug therapy for this condition should not be done in primary care, but should be carried out in a secondary care setting. The suggested role of primary care is that of engaging with and supporting the patients and their carers while also reviewing the patient and the medications used. There is an emphasis on lithium only being started by secondary care unless a shared care agreement is in place with secondary care. The same applies to valproate.

Pharmacological interventions

Initial management

Initial management of an acute episode of mania or hypomania is with antipsychotic drugs. Haloperidol, olanzapine, quetiapine or risperidone are recommended. It is recommended that, where possible, any antidepressant medication the patient may be on is stopped. If the initial antipsychotic medication is poorly tolerated at any dose, or is ineffective at the maximum licensed dose then an alternative from the above list should be offered. If this is also ineffective the consideration should be given to the addition of lithium. If this is unsuitable, usually due to patient preference, or it is ineffective consider adding in valproate.

Benzodiazepines such as lorazepam can be used in the treatment of a person in the initial stages. They can be useful to help manage some of the behavioural changes such as agitation that may be seen. They should only be used for a very short time due to their propensity to cause addiction.

Prophylaxis

Lithium or valproate may be used as prophylactic treatment in patients with previous episodes of bipolar disorder. However, if mania develops in these patients antipsychotic medications should be initiated. Watch these patients closely as they will be prone to developing depression. Monitor the plasma lithium levels in patients on lithium as it has a narrow therapeutic window and this will allow optimization of the dose and thus the treatment.

In a patient with severe mania that has not responded to medication electroconvulsive therapy may be considered.

Depression management

The management of moderate to severe depression in a patient with bipolar disorder is initially with a combination of fluoxetine and olanzapine or the use of quetiapine on its own depending on which is tolerated and acceptable to the patient. Treatment with olanzapine alone can also be considered if the patient prefers, as can lamotrigine alone. Lamotrigine should also be considered if there is no response to fluoxetine and olanzapine or quetiapine on its own.

If the patient is already on valproate, ensure that the dose is optimal prior to adding in the further treatments outlined above.

Long-term management

Once the patient is stable and the acute episode has been effectively treated long-term treatment with mood stabilizing drugs should be considered.

Lithium is the drug of choice for the prevention of relapse. However, it does require regular blood testing to ensure the plasma concentration stays within the therapeutic window. If lithium is ineffective or not acceptable to the patient, consider adding in valproate or using it as a single agent. Olanzapine or quetiapine may also be used depending on the patient's previous response to these medications.

Specific guidance is offered by NICE (2014) about the use of the different classes of medication. Although some of this has been dealt with previously it is worth going over again.

Before starting antipsychotic medication record baseline figures for weight (or body mass index), pulse, blood pressure, fasting blood glucose (or HbA_{1c}) and a lipid profile. If the product profile suggests it or if there is a patient history of potential cardiac risk factors do an ECG (remember all inpatients should have an ECG on admission).

Treat the commencement of any antipsychotic medication as a therapeutic trial. Discuss and record what side-effects the patient is willing to put up with. Record the indications for treatment, the expected outcomes and side-effects, and the timescales involved. Use appropriate doses of medication and do not exceed the recommended maximum dose in the BNF except in exceptional circumstances. If a dose beyond the recommended dose is used record your justification for doing so. Make sure the patient is aware of the unlicensed use of medication where it occurs. Record your reasons for changing or stopping medications and any responses that may occur because of these changes.

Pulse and blood pressure should be monitored at every dose change. In practical terms it may make more sense to build this into your standard examination at every visit. Weight should be recorded weekly for the first 6 weeks and then at 12 weeks and annually after that. Monitoring of blood glucose and lipid profile should be carried out at 12 weeks and then annually after that. Remember to check for movement disorders at every review. Also record side-effects and response to treatment. Also attempt to assess adherence to the treatment regimen.

When looking at starting lithium you should make sure that the patient understands that concordance with this medication is critical. A failure of concordance runs an increased risk of the reoccurrence of symptoms. Prior to starting the lithium baseline measurements of body mass index, urea and electrolytes, estimated glomerular filtration rate, thyroid function, full blood count and bone group are needed. If indicated an ECG should be done.

Plasma lithium levels should be measured one week after initiating therapy then weekly until the level is stable. If there is a change in dose the level should be rechecked one week after the dose changes. Initially the aim is to maintain a level of between 0.6 and 0.8mmol/l. However, if there has been a relapse or symptoms have not fully settled a higher plasma concentration of 0.8 to 1.0mmol/l should be maintained for at least six months before the dose is lowered with a view to obtaining the lower plasma concentration range outlined above.

The patient needs to be aware that they need to seek urgent review if they develop diarrhoea or vomiting. Or if they become physically acutely unwell. Fluid balance is also critical and needs to be maintained. If there is any excessive fluid loss, say through excess sweating or fever, fluid intake should be increased accordingly. People on lithium should be warned that they should not take non-steroidal anti-inflammatory drugs.

Once stable, the lithium level should be checked every three months for the first year then every six months. There are exceptions to this and three monthly monitoring should be continued in patients who are older, who are on drugs that interact with lithium, those with a reduced estimated glomerular filtration rates or thyroid function, or those with raised calcium levels. This should also be continued in those patients with poor concordance, poor symptom control or those who are maintained in the higher plasma concentration range.

In stable patients, repeating the body mass index and the baseline bloods every six months will suffice. However, you should increase the frequency of testing if there is any impairment or irregularity noted.

Watch out for any signs of neurotoxicity. These include cognitive impairment, ataxia, paraesthesia and tremor. This may be seen at blood levels over 1mmol/l but is more common at levels over 1.5mmol/l.

When initiating treatment with sodium valproate make sure that there are baseline recordings of body mass index, fasting blood sugar and liver function. Educate the patient and their carers about the signs and symptoms of liver disease and of haematological disorders. Advise them to seek urgent medical review if any of these symptoms present. If any blood dyscrasia is detected or if there is evidence of abnormal liver function valproate should be stopped at once. Be aware and make the patient and carers aware of the interactions of valproate with other anti-epileptic medication and also with smoking.

Repeating the baseline measurements every six months is important, but there is only a place for measuring valproate levels if it is ineffective, there is poor concordance or toxicity. This should not be done routinely. Signs of toxicity include tremor, lethargy and disturbances in gait. Be particularly vigilant for these in elderly patients.

Do not use valproate in women of childbearing age. This is because of effects that can be seen on a developing foetus.

Prior to starting a patient on lamotrigine record baseline full blood count, liver function and urea and electrolytes tests. Follow the instructions on starting this medication as laid out in the BNF. Remember that there are adverse interactions between lamotrigine and valproate that should be considered in patients already on valproate. Patients and carers should be told to seek urgent medical review if the patient develops a rash. Review is also needed if they become pregnant or are considering becoming pregnant.

Do not measure lamotrigine levels unless there is toxicity or poor concordance.

For further reading on the management guideline for this condition please look at NICE guidelines (CG185, NICE, 2014).

Pharmacology of mood stabilizers

Some of the medications we have looked at above are discussed in other chapters as their use in mania is not their main licensing indication or use. We will discuss here the drugs for which bipolar effective disorders is the main indication or where we do not cover the drug in other chapters.

Lithium

Lithium has for many years been the mainstay of mood stabilizing medication used in these disorders. It continues to be used and you will see many patients for whom this is their main or only medication. It is used in the form of lithium salts and more than one form is available. Lithium carbonate is the most commonly used but lithium citrate is also used.

Its chemical effects are many and once lithium is in the blood it can have an effect at many receptor and neurotransmitter systems. As it has many interactions its exact medicinal action on mania is not known. The drug has a narrow therapeutic index and this means that if not taken in the correct way the blood levels can move out of the plasma range necessary for therapeutic effect. Below the required level the drug becomes ineffective, so it is important that patients do not miss doses. Above the required level it becomes toxic and the patient can suffer harmful side-effects and even adverse effects related to the high levels of the drug in the blood. Lithium overdoses can be fatal. Side-effects at normal doses are rare but nystagmus has been reported in some patients. Some extra-pyramidal effects have been noted (see Chapter 8). Due to this narrow therapeutic window, you need to be aware that there are other physiological circumstances that can lead the patient to have higher than normal plasma levels and to show signs of toxicity. Patients should be advised that dehydration can increase lithium levels and that remaining adequately hydrated while on lithium therapy is important. Interaction with other medications can lead to changes in plasma levels of lithium so careful review of medication before commencement of therapy is important.

Symptoms of lithium toxicity to look for are:

- nausea, vomiting and diarrhoea;
- ataxia;
- confusion;
- lethargy;
- abnormal reflexes;
- nystagmus;
- renal impairment in severe toxicity;
- convulsions in severe toxicity.

Sudden death can occur if signs of toxicity are not spotted and acted upon promptly. If a patient reports the symptoms above, the plasma level should be checked and the patient admitted for observation.

Sodium valproate

This drug, now used as a mood stabilizer, belongs to the drug class of antiepileptics and was (and still is) used in the management of epilepsy. It is most useful in patients for whom mania is the predominant phase of their disorder. It can also be used in patients in remission to prevent relapse into either a depressive or manic phase. Although, like lithium, its exact mechanism of action is not understood, we know that it has some effect at GABA receptors by increasing the levels of GABAergic transmission leading to overall inhibitory effects in neuronal activity within the brain. This is the proposed main effect in its ability as an anticonvulsant and it is possible that this inhibitory effect could contribute to its use in mood stabilization.

It is also associated with side-effects but unlike lithium its risk in overdose is substantially less of a problem and as such measures such as frequent and regular plasma level checks are not required. This gives sodium valproate an advantage over lithium from a patient perspective. Side-effects include gastrointestinal disturbances that can be minor, weight gain, transient hair loss (regrowth can be thick and curly) and rarely blood dyscrasias are seen along with some cognitive impairment.

It should not be used in pregnancy and should be avoided in women of childbearing age unless contraception is guaranteed – although even then it should be avoided as it has been linked with the development of polycystic ovarian syndrome. If given in pregnancy it is associated with significantly higher than normal birth anomalies including spina bifida, developmental delay, autism and rarely valproate syndrome.

It is important that you gain a working familiarity with these medications used in practice. You should be able to use the BNF to look up the medicines and to ascertain any effects and side-effects your patients may experience. You should also be able to use Appendix One of the BNF to check for interactions that these medications may have with other medications your patient may be taking at the same time.

Key learning points

Bipolar affective disorder

▶ Bipolar affective disorder is characterized by 'swings' of mood from mania to depression.
▶ Other forms of mood disorder such as mania and hypomania also occur.
▶ Sufferers can have predominance of one mood over the other but both must be present for the diagnosis to be made.

Physiology and pharmacology

▶ The exact cause of bipolar affective disorder is unknown but it is thought to involve biological, psychological, social and environmental factors.
▶ Treatment can include management of acute episodes of mania or depression or can involve prophylactic management of a patient in remission to prevent relapse to either end of the mood spectrum.
▶ Medication such as lithium and sodium valproate have been shown to be effective mood stabilizers.
▶ Antipsychotic medication can be used in the management of manic episodes.
▶ Antidepressant medication can be used in the management of depressive episodes.

Drug calculations

1 Your patient requires 500mg of valproate three times a day. You have 250mg tablets.

How many tablets for one dose?

How many tablets for one day?

2 Your patient requires 1g of lithium carbonate daily. You have 250mg tablets.

How many tablets per day?

How many tablets for a seven-day supply?

3 Your patient requires 509mg of lithium citrate daily. You have 101.8mg in 1ml solution.

How many ml per day?

How many ml for a seven-day supply?

$\longrightarrow$

←

4 Your patient requires lithium carbonate 400mg daily. He has been prescribed a box of 100 × 200mg tablets.

How long will this prescription last them?

5 Your patient requires valproate 750mg daily. You have 150mg tablets.

How many tablets per day?

How many tablets for a 28-day supply?

6 Your patient requires 509mg of lithium citrate twice daily. You have 203.6mg in 1ml solution.

How many ml per dose?

How many ml per day?

How many ml for a 28-day supply?

7 Your patient requires lithium citrate 3.12g per day in two divided doses. You have a 150ml bottle of 104mg in 1ml solution.

How long will this bottle last the patient?

8 Your patient requires 900mg of lithium carbonate modified-release tablets daily. You have a box of 60 × 450mg tablets.

How long will this box last your patient?

9 Your patient requires 1g of lithium carbonate daily. You have 200mg tablets. The box of 100 tablets costs £2.20.

What is the cost of a 28-day supply at this price?

10 Your patient requires 1.018g of lithium citrate daily. You have a 150ml bottle of 101.8mg in 1ml solution. This costs £5.79.

How much does a 30-day supply of this medicine cost at this price?

Multiple choice questions

Try answering these multiple choice questions to test what you have learned from reading this chapter. You can check your answers on page 154.

1 The drug lithium is described as a

   a) Mood stabilizer
   b) Mood enhancer
   c) Mood leveller
   d) Mood altering drug

→

←

2 Sodium valproate is a drug now commonly used in bipolar affective disorder. What was it initially used for as a main indication?

a) Depression
b) Hypertension
c) Epilepsy
d) Diabetes

3 Patients on lithium should have what monitored regularly?

a) Electroencephalogram (EEG)
b) Blood levels
c) Computed tomography scan
d) Urinalysis

4 Antipsychotic drugs should be used

a) As first-line treatment for all mania-related disorders
b) In acute episodes of mania
c) As long-term management of hypomania
d) For all of the above

5 What blood levels would constitute an overdose of lithium?

a) >0.5mmols/l
b) >0.75mmols/l
c) >1.0mmols/l
d) >1.5mmols/l

6 What is the number of the NICE guideline involved in the management of bipolar disorder?

a) CG195
b) CG95
c) CG185
d) CG102

7 What was bipolar disorder previously referred to as?

a) Manic state
b) Hypomania
c) Manic psychosis
d) Manic depression

→

8 Commencement of initial drug therapy after diagnosis should occur

  a) In primary care
  b) In secondary care
  c) Supervised by a psychiatrist
  d) In a shared care agreement

9 When can benzodiazepines be used in mania?

  a) Long-term management
  b) Short-term management of a depressive disorder
  c) Initial stages of treatment for agitation
  d) Never

10 After initiating lithium therapy, how soon should you monitor plasma levels?

  a) One hour
  b) One day
  c) One week
  d) One month

Case study

Mr Khan is a 55-year-old highly successful banker. He has suffered from bipolar affective disorder since his early 20s and had been managed well on lithium of varying doses since then. He has had manic episodes in the past but has always managed to restabilize on his lithium. He has read about valproate as an alternative to lithium and wishes to discuss the possibility of changing medication. Discuss the options that can be outlined to Mr Khan.

Recommended websites

British National Formulary (BNF): www.bnf.org
EMC medicines compendium: www.medicines.org.uk

Recommended further reading

National Institute for Health and Care Excellence (NICE) (2014) *Bipolar Disorder: Assessment and Management. CG185.* London: NICE. Available at: https://www.nice.org.uk/guidance/cg185 (accessed 23 February 2016).

Royal College of Psychiatrists (2012) *Bipolar affective Disorder (Manic Depression): Information for Parents, Carers and Anyone who Works with Young People.* London: Royal College of Psychiatrists. Available at: http://www.rcpsych.ac.uk/healthadvice/parentsandyouthinfo/parentscarers/bipolaraffectivedisorder.aspx (accessed 23 February 2016).

World Health Organization (WHO) (2016) *International Statistical Classification of Diseases and Related Health Problems 10th Revision (ICD-10) – WHO Version for 2016.* Available at: http://apps.who.int/classifications/icd10/browse/2016/en (accessed 19 February 2016).

Substance misuse: drugs, alcohol and legal highs

11

Chapter contents

Learning objectives

After reading this chapter you will have gained knowledge around:

- The incidence of substance misuse in the UK.
- The legal frameworks governing the control and supply of drugs of abuse.
- The misuse of prescribed and over-the-counter medications.
- The pharmacodynamic actions of drugs used in the management of substance misuse.

Introduction

There are a number of drugs susceptible to misuse. Some are more readily regarded as food stuffs, some are prescribed but most are illicit. The ICD-10 criteria (WHO 2016) breaks them down into nine basic categories. These are alcohol, opiates, cannabis, sedatives, cocaine, stimulants (including caffeine), hallucinogens, tobacco and volatile solvents. There is also a recognition that these are often used, with or without intent, in combination. Also it should be recognized that, given the inventiveness of the world's young amateur chemists, this list cannot be viewed as exhaustive.

The use of a substance passes through a number of stages on the way to addiction. Initially there is acute intoxication. This occurs in the period immediately after ingestion of the substance. It is characterized by changes in the levels of cognition and consciousness. It may also affect thoughts, feelings and behaviour. The degree of intoxication is often, but not always, dose related. This can be complicated by habituation or by concomitant physical disease such as liver disease or renal impairment. Acute intoxication is transient and the degree of intoxication should lessen as the length of time since ingestion increases.

Recurrent drug use may result in damaging consequences. When there is an associated effect on physical, social or mental health the drug use might be described as harmful. Harmful drug use is often recognized by others and may lead to adverse social consequences.

Dependence occurs when drug-seeking behaviour becomes of greater importance to the individual than the tasks normally associated with daily living, for example when 'scoring' is more important than going to work. This behaviour is characterized by the following.

- A strong desire to take the substance.
- Difficulty controlling where, when, and how much is taken.
- A requirement to take greater doses to obtain the same effect.
- Evidence of psychological withdrawal symptoms if the drug is stopped.

- A decline in other behaviours that had previously been pleasurable.
- Continuing use of the drug despite obvious damage being done to the patient's physical or mental wellbeing and their social standing.

There is a need to understand the drug's pharmacology and the physical and psychological effects of its use as well as having an understanding of the withdrawal symptoms associated with stopping the drug. Different substances produce different withdrawal symptoms with differences in the potential risks associated with stopping the drug.

There is more information available on this that goes beyond the remit of this chapter but if you are interested then consider looking at the ICD-10 mental health sections F10–F19 (WHO 2016). Let us now consider the incidence of substance misuse.

Prevalence and incidence of substance misuse

Statistics and data are published on known levels of drug and substance misuse by the Health and Social Care Information Centre (2014). The data relating to England in 2014 (which was published in December 2014 and is the latest published data available at the time of writing) was published based on the information held about drug misuse in the adult and child population. This information was gathered from a variety of sources and included admissions to hospital as a result of drug misuse. It is, however, data about *known* misuse only and there is probably a hidden group of drug misusers, not known to any relevant agency, so these figures are representative but not exhaustive. The data relates to the years 2013–2014 and it is not broken down by drug name. The data are summarized in Box 11.1 (Health and Social Care Information Centre 2014).

The Home Office (2014) also publishes data on drug misuse and they take their findings from the crime survey from England and Wales. For the same period (2013–2014) they produced the following key facts:

Box 11.1 Drug misuse data

Drug misuse among adults

In England and Wales in 2013/14:

- Around 1 in 11 adults aged 16–59 (8.8 per cent) had taken an illicit drug in the past year. However, this proportion more than doubled when looking at the age subgroup of 16- to 24-year-olds (18.9 per cent). These figures are an increase from 2012/13 when 8.1 per cent of 16- to 59-year-olds and 16.2 per cent of 16- to 24-year-olds had taken an illicit drug in the past year. However, both figures are lower than they were in 1996.

Drug misuse among children (11–15 years)

In England in 2013:

- 16 per cent of pupils had ever taken drugs, 11 per cent had taken them in the past year and 6 per cent had taken them in the past month. This is similar to the levels of drug use recorded in 2011 and 2012. However, between 2003 and 2011 drug use among 11- to 15-year-olds declined.

Health outcomes

In England in 2013/14:

- There were 7104 admissions to hospital with a primary diagnosis of a drug-related mental health and behavioural disorder. This is an increase of 8.5 per cent (555 admissions) from 2012/13 when there were 6549 such admissions. Overall, between 2003/04 and 2013/14 admissions have decreased by 11 per cent (765) from 7869 to 7104.
- There were 13,917 admissions with a primary diagnosis of poisoning by illicit drugs. Overall, there has been a 76.7 per cent (6041) increase since 2003/04 when there were 7876 such admissions.
- There were 1957 deaths related to misuse of illicit drugs in 2013, an increase of 321 from 2012 when there were 1636 such deaths. This is contrary to the downward trend since 2008 when deaths peaked at 2004.

- Cocaine, Ecstasy, LSD (lysergic acid diethylamide) and ketamine use increased between 2012/13 and 2013/14. However, there were no statistically significant decreases in past year drug use of any individual drug types among 16- to 59-year-olds between 2012/13 and 2013/14.
- Around one-third of adults had taken drugs at some point during their lifetime. Of 16- to 59-year-olds, 35.6% had reported ever using drugs.

These figures correlate with the ones presented above and suggest that the picture we get from crime surveys and additional sources gives a fairly accurate account of detectable substance misuse of known and illegal substances. It does not, however, give us a picture around the use of legal highs, a new and worrying area of substance misuse. This will be discussed in more detail later in this chapter.

Legal frameworks around drugs of abuse

The most important pieces of legislation that control the availability of psychoactive drugs in the UK are discussed now.

The Medicines Act 1968

- Controls the production and supply of medicinal products.
- Its main purpose is to protect the public from harm, that is, to ensure as far as possible that medicinal products are safe and effective.
- Identifies practitioners that have the authority to prescribe.
- This restricts the availability of medicines by classifying them as:
  - general sales list: GSL;
  - pharmacy medicines: P;
  - prescription-only medicines: POM.

It is an act of parliament so its contents are laid down in statute law. It governs *who, where* and *in what circumstances* medicine can be *prescribed, stored, supplied and administered* in the UK. Any activity that goes outside any of those areas is a breach of the Medicines Act and this is a criminal offence. Any infringement would be subject to criminal proceedings and the person committing the infringement may face a fine or even imprisonment.

This applies to *all* medicinal products with some exceptions around herbal remedies and it covers medicines intended for human and veterinary use.

Amendments have been made to the Act over the years but the Act of 1968 is the standing legislation. Most notable examples of amendments are the addition of nurses, pharmacists and certain allied health professionals, giving them the status of appropriate practitioner under the Act, which allowed for the advancement of non-medical prescribing practice in the UK.

The Misuse of Drugs Act 1971

This Act categorized psychoactive drugs into classes that are not directly relevant to pharmaceutical practice but which are used in law.

As well as governing supply, the Misuse of Drugs Act (1971) also deals with possession. It outlines the criminal offences under which convictions are usually made and divides drugs into one of three groups:

- Class A;
- Class B;
- Class C.

Penalties are imposed according to the offence, class of drug and quantity involved. Previous convictions are also taken into consideration. The Misuse of Drugs Act classification and penalties associated with common substances are summarized in Table 11.1.

Note that the legal position on 'magic mushrooms' will depend whether the mushroom species in question contains any active substance controlled by the Misuse of Drugs Act and may also depend on whether the mushrooms are prepared for consumption or not.

In January 2004 cannabis was reclassified from Class B to C. This meant that if someone over 18 was found in possession of a small amount of cannabis for personal use they would have been unlikely to be arrested. Instead, the drug would be confiscated and they would be cautioned. If the person was caught repeatedly they may well have been arrested and charged, particularly if caught in a public place. However, this was reversed by the Home Office in 2009 and cannabis remains in category B with the attendant regulation and enforcement that goes with it.

Although the Misuse of Drugs Act sets out the main categories and penalties as seen above there are further regulations that also need to be considered.

Table 11.1 Classification of some commonly misused substances

Class	Drugs	Maximum penalties
A	Cocaine including crack cocaine, diamorphine, dipipanone, Ecstasy, LSD (lysergic acid diethylamide), methadone, morphine, opium, pethidine	Seven years imprisonment and/or unlimited fine for possession. Life imprisonment and/or fine for supply
B	Most amphetamines, cannabis, codeine and dihydrocodeine, methylphenidate	Five years imprisonment and/or fine for possession. Fourteen years imprisonment and a fine for supply
C	Benzodiazepines, anabolic steroids and growth hormones	Two years imprisonment and/or fine for possession. Five years imprisonment and/or fine for supply

Adapted from the Misuse of Drugs Act 1971

The Misuse of Drugs Regulations 2001

These place further restraint on controlled drugs (CD) relating to medical and pharmaceutical practice by placing them in different 'schedules' which determine how they are obtained, stored and supplied. These schedules are the ones relevant to all prescribing and administration and also to pharmacists' safe storage and dispensing practice. There are five schedules.

- *Schedule 1* (CD Lic): includes the hallucinogenic drugs (for example LSD) and Ecstasy-type substances that have virtually no therapeutic use and includes cannabis, mescaline and psilocin. A Home Office Licence is required to possess these drugs legally.
- *Schedule 2* (CD POM): includes the opiates (such as morphine and diamorphine), and the major stimulants (such as amphetamines). It also includes quinalbarbitone, methadone and codeine and dihydrocodeine. Safe custody requirements apply to all Schedule 2 drugs.
- *Schedule 3* (CD No Register): minor stimulant drugs, temazepam, phenobarbitone, buprenorphine etc.
- *Schedule 4* (CD Benz) and (CD Anab): includes most of the benzodiazepines and anabolic/androgenic steroids.
- *Schedule 5* (CD Inv): includes products that contain a controlled drug but only in low strength, for example, co-codamol, co-dydramol etc.

A number of amendments to the Misuse of Drugs Regulations 2001 came into force on the 14 November 2005. These included the following.

- A removal of the handwriting requirement for controlled drug prescriptions. Prescriptions can now be computer generated and only the signature needs to be handwritten.
- Computerized controlled drugs registers are now allowed.
- Extended formulary nurse prescribers are permitted to prescribe a wider range of controlled drugs in specific circumstances.
- Ascorbic acid has been added to the list of drug paraphernalia that can be supplied to illicit drug users for the administration or preparation of controlled drugs, as part of drug treatment programmes.

Further amendments were made in 2012 to allow prescription of controlled drugs in schedules 2–5 to be carried out by independent pharmacist and nurse prescribers. In 2015 a small list of certain controlled drugs was made available to independent physiotherapist and podiatrist prescribers.

It is also prudent for us to consider legislation around the effects that consuming psychoactive substances can have on our ability to drive a car or other vehicle.

The Road Traffic Act 1988

This act makes it illegal to be in charge of a motor vehicle if 'unfit to drive through drink or drugs'. This includes illicit and prescribed medicines. This act requires drivers to notify the Driving and Vehicle Licensing Agency (DVLA) if there is any reason that the safety of their driving may be impaired, including disability, by the misuse of drugs or the receipt of a prescription for drugs that impair reactions or cause sedation. The responsibility for notification to the DVLA lies with the patient not healthcare professionals although it may be necessary for a medical professional to disclose relevant information to the medical adviser at the DVLA if a patient continues to drive when they may not be fit to do so. The Act also allows the police to test for impairment to drive due to drugs and/or alcohol.

Legal highs and over-the-counter/prescribed medications

Legal highs

Legal highs can encompass a range of medicines or substances that have the primary action of having a psychoactive effect similar to other drugs or substances of misuse such as cocaine and Ecstasy, two drugs that are, of course, illegal. More and more substances seem to be becoming available and are often marketed as legal highs or sold as substances for other purposes (not for human consumption) to get around the law. Research in this area has been limited and the knowledge we have around the dangers of these substances is scant. Research is being carried out into some of these legal highs that are becoming more common to see if they should be made illegal. It is prudent to assume that a substance that has psycho active properties should not be considered safe just because it is legal.

These legal highs can take many forms. Some are sold in powder formulation but some are made into tablets or capsules for ease of administration. Others are in a state (or are made into formulations) that are intended to be smoked. They are usually marketed in colourful and eye-catching packaging and their labelling does not give a true indication of their content. It is difficult to know therefore exactly what is being consumed. This in itself is an inherent danger.

The range of effects that can be derived from legal highs is similar to that of their illegal counterparts. Some have a stimulant activity – the so called 'uppers'. Some have sedative properties – the 'downers'. And some possess activity that renders hallucinogenic effect. Legal highs are very often taken by people who are already under the influence of other drugs and/or alcohol. As we have virtually no data on these substances it goes without saying that we have even less information on their interaction. This is a growing area of concern, and of research, and it is anticipated that some legal highs will be made illegal or at least be subject to some regulation. Management of patients admitted after taking legal highs remains problematic as the contents of the substance are often not known and treatment is contained to symptom management.

Of course, we have to consider and acknow ledge the misuse of legally available substances such as alcohol and tobacco, as much of the work done in healthcare is around management of harmful drinking and smoking cessation. Smoking cessation will not be covered here, but we will consider the management of problem drinking.

Alcohol-use disorder

Alcohol-use disorder is a diagnosis given when problem drinking becomes severe. The drinking should have been problematic for a long period of time and the person drinking should be suffering from symptoms that indicate severe dependence on the alcohol, as well as debilitating symptoms from the misuse. These include:

- drinking more or for longer;
- an inability to cut down or stop drinking despite successive attempts;
- memory blackouts;
- absence from work due to drinking behaviour;
- risk-taking behaviour or criminal activity;
- withdrawal symptoms from alcohol such as:
  - tremor
  - restlessness
  - nausea
  - sweating
  - palpitations
  - seizure.

Alcohol-use disorder is a recognized problem within our society and it is not restricted to particular age, social or demographic groups. Its diagnosis, assessment and treatment falls largely under mental health services in the UK.

Prescription medications

It has long been known that some medications available by prescription have the potential to be abused, or cause tolerance and dependence. The prescribing of these medications is to some extent controlled and regulated by the legislation we looked at above; however, misuse of prescription medications does still occur.

Certain prescribed medications are known to be subject to higher levels of misuse than others. These include:

- codeine and dihydrocodeine;
- morphine and diamorphine;
- methadone;
- benzodiazepines;
- barbiturates;
- hypnotics;
- stimulant medications.

The reason that people misuse prescription medications can be multifactorial. Some misuse is indirect or unintentional, some is down to the properties of the drug themselves causing tolerance and sometimes it is direct and wilful misuse. Whatever the reason early detection and intervention is required to manage the problem before it escalates.

Pharmacological interventions and management

Management of substance abuse

In view of the many different potential substances of abuse it is important to start with the shared principles of management. First, the aim of managing patients with substance abuse is harm reduction. That is not only the harm that the drug addiction may be doing to the patient, but also the potential harm that the addicted patient may be wreaking on society. For example methadone replacement therapy used to manage opiate addiction not only allows the patient to stabilize and address their health issues, but also by removing the need of the patient to finance their drug habit it may also reduce the crime rate in that area.

In all addiction management strategies there is an emphasis on supportive and talking therapies. This allows the identification of concomitant needs whether they are disease related, such as associated depression, renal and liver disease or HIV, or social needs such as housing, finance or support in the workplace. It also allows the patient to be educated as to what to expect from the withdrawal process and provides the support needed to allow the patient to progress through this period of withdrawal and stabilization.

During the process of withdrawal there may be the need to treat potentially dangerous issues caused by the drug withdrawal; an example of this would be the management of *delirium tremens* in patients withdrawing from alcohol. In other cases replacement therapies may be offered and either maintained, as often happens with methadone, or gradually reduced, as happens with nicotine patches in patients trying to stop smoking. It is essential to continue supporting patients through this stage as well.

Box 11.2 Variations in guidelines and services

It is important to recognize at this point that although there are national guidelines for managing many of the drugs of addiction, most trusts have derived local guidelines from these and there may be differences in both the guidelines being used from trust to trust, but also in the services that have been commissioned to manage these patients. Many areas have specialist services to deal with opiate, nicotine and alcohol addiction, but may leave to the local primary care teams the management of addictions to cocaine, LSD, amphetamines and other drugs, where there is a less pharmacological approach to treatment.

Drugs used in smoking cessation include various forms of nicotine replacement therapies, varenicline and bupropion. The use of these drugs and the protocols that go with them can be found in the NICE guidelines: *PH10: Stop Smoking Services* (2008).

Drugs used in the management of alcohol-use disorders include diazepam, chlordiazepoxide, acamprosate, naltrexone and disulfiram. The protocols for their use can be found in NICE *CG115* (2011), which looks at management of alcohol-use disorders, in conjunction with NICE *CG100* (2010), which addresses physical complications of alcohol-use disorders.

Methadone, buprenorphine, lofexidine and naltrexone are drugs used in the management of opiate addiction. Guidance for the use of these drugs and the management of opiate and benzodiazepine addiction can be found in the Department of Health document *Drug Misuse and Dependence: UK Guidelines on Clinical Management* (this is from 2007 but is currently under review).

Remember that local protocols will exist for the management of many of these conditions and that these would be worth reviewing.

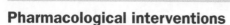

Pharmacological interventions

It is worth explaining that although the aim of the treatments outlined above remains the case for all substance misuse interventions, there are different ways of approaching the pharmacological management. These fall into three broad categories:

- reduction therapy;
- replacement therapy;
- management of abstinence.

Even when pharmacological management is required, it is important to remember that psychosocial interventions should also be implemented. But for now the three pharmacological management approaches will be explored in more detail.

Reduction therapy

This is most useful when dealing with misuse of prescribed medication where the prescriber can, in a controlled and systematic manner, reduce the amount of the prescribed medication over a defined period of time with regular review and monitoring. It involves prescribing the same drug the patient is misusing in gradually smaller amounts. The hope in doing this is that any withdrawal symptoms, physical or psychological, can be mitigated and controlled. It is important to monitor for, and therefore be aware of, the withdrawal symptoms that can be expected.

Replacement therapy

This is a common form of prescribing in drug misuse of substances such as opiates and in smoking cessation. The principle is to replace the harmful substance with one that is deemed 'safer' to mitigate against withdrawal. The use of methadone in opiate addiction is a good example. Methadone is a legally prescribable synthetic opioid drug that can be given in monitored and controlled doses to prevent the person continuing with drug-seeking behaviour and the risk taking that is often associated with opiate addiction. The methadone dose will be titrated to match the effect the user was achieving from their opiate. It acts at the same opioid receptors in the body as their drug of misuse and has an effect of pharmacological mimicry. Supervised consumption forms part of the programme of treatment. Once stabilization has occurred it is possible for the patient to move to reduction therapy as outlined above as they would now be transferred, on a legally prescribable medication, to where this can be facilitated by non-medical prescribing healthcare professionals.

Management of abstinence and withdrawal

For some cases of substance misuse, the two interventions above are either inappropriate or have been ineffective. Sometimes a course of action of managed abstinence is undertaken, whereby the patient abstains from the drug of addiction but, due to the emergence of withdrawal symptoms, requires that abstinence period to be managed with pharmacological intervention. An example of this is the prescribing that is undertaken in patients with alcohol-use disorder when they stop drinking and in the removal of opiates without reduction or replacement.

Opiate withdrawal

Patients may exhibit many signs of withdrawal related to the removal of opiates. These are summarized in Table 11.2.

Some of these signs and symptoms can be managed with psychological interventions, but some of the physical symptoms may be severe enough to require pharmacological intervention. It would be appropriate to manage severe diarrhoea by prescribing loperamide. It is also appropriate to mitigate some of the symptoms by prescription of lofexidine. This is a non-opioid drug with actions at adrenergic receptors and is effective in reducing the physical symptoms. It is licensed and authorized for the management of opiate withdrawal.

Other medications that have been used in withdrawal from opiates are non-steroidal anti-inflammatory drugs or mebeverine for management of muscle cramps and short-term benzodiazepines for help with sleep disturbance. If nausea and vomiting is a significant problem then metoclopramide or prochlorperazine can be used.

Alcohol withdrawal

This is an important area of prescribing as the signs and symptoms of alcohol withdrawal

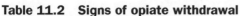

Table 11.2   Signs of opiate withdrawal

Objective and measurable signs	Subjective signs
Yawning	Restlessness
Coughing and or sneezing	Irritability
Runny nose and/or eyes	Anxiety
Raised pulse and/or blood pressure	Sleep disturbance
Dilated pupils	Depressive symptoms
Clamminess	Cravings
Diarrhoea and nausea/vomiting	
Muscle tremor and cramps	

(sometimes grouped into the term *delirium tremens* or 'DTs') can be serious and sometimes even fatal. Let us just recap on the typical symptoms of alcohol withdrawal, which include:

- tremor;
- restlessness;
- nausea;
- sweating;
- palpitations;
- seizure.

There are many medications that can be used in alcohol withdrawal and these are summarized here.

- Chlordiazepoxide – this is a long-acting benzodiazepine and is used routinely in assisted withdrawal. It has classical benzodiazepine effects as described in Chapter 6 (anxiety). It is helpful in symptom control as it can suppress many of the symptoms outlined above.
- Acamprosate is useful for patients who have withdrawn from alcohol and it can prevent relapse. Treatment should commence as soon as abstinence has been achieved and continue for one year.
- Disulfiram is given to help achieve abstinence. When taken, if alcohol is imbibed while on this drug an extreme and unpleasant reaction occurs. It is for this reason it is sometimes referred to as aversion therapy. Symptoms occur within 10–20 minutes of consuming alcohol and are brought about by the accumulation

of acetaldehyde, which provokes flushing, headache, palpitations, nausea and vomiting. It is only effective if taken on a daily basis.

- Vitamin supplements – administration of certain vitamins is recommended in management of alcohol-use disorders. Patients who are dependent on alcohol can be deficient in certain nutritional factors such as thiamine and folic acid. Replacement of these can prevent the development of Wernicke Syndrome and encephalopathy.
- Naltrexone – this drug is an opioid receptor antagonist found to have benefit in prevention of relapse after successful alcohol withdrawal.

It is important that you gain a working familiarity with these medications used in practice and also the medications that are being misused by the patients and clients you are working with. You should be able to use the BNF to look up the medicines discussed and to ascertain any effects and side-effects your patients may experience. You may need to use other sources such as some of the websites suggested at the end of this chapter to look for information around the illegal substances that are being misused. You should also be able to use Appendix One of the BNF to check for interactions that these medications may have with other medications your patient may be taking at the same time. It is to be remembered though that due to the nature or unknown nature of many legal highs, the ability to check for interactions in these cases will be limited or perhaps even impossible.

Key learning points

Substance misuse

▶ Substance misuse and abuse is widespread and problematic in the UK.
▶ Substances that are misused vary and include illegal substances, legal highs, prescription medications, alcohol and tobacco.
▶ People who misuse substances come from all social, cultural, age and demographic backgrounds.

Legislation

▶ There is a variety of legislation concerning the prescription, supply and administration of medications.
▶ Separate legislation exists for medications that are deemed to be controlled substances.
▶ Nurses should be familiar with the legislation around prescribed medication.

Pharmacology

▶ Pharmacological intervention may be appropriate in conjunction with psychosocial approaches.
▶ Pharmacological intervention can be reduction based, replacement based or managed abstinence based.

Drug calculations

1 Your patient requires 500mg of disulfiram daily. You have 200mg scored tablets.

How many tablets per day?

How many tablets for a 28-day supply?

2 Your patient requires a weekly dose of naltrexone 350mg to be given over three days in the week, 150mg one day and 100mg on the other two days. You have 50mg tablets.

How many tablets for day one?

How many tablets daily for day two and day three?

How many tablets per week?

How many tablets for a 28-day supply?

3 Your patient requires lofexidine 800mg daily in two divided doses. You have 200mg tablets.

How many tablets per dose?

How many tablets per day?

How many tablets for a 28-day supply?

4 Your patient requires methadone 30mg daily. You have 5mg tablets.

How many tablets per day?

5 Your patient requires methadone 120mg daily. You have 20mg per ml oral solution.

How many ml per day?

6 Your patient requires chlordiazepoxide 30mg four times a day. You have 10mg capsules.

How many capsules per dose?

How many capsules per day?

7 Your patient requires loperamide 4mg twice daily. You have 200 micrograms in 1ml solution.

How many ml per dose?

How many ml per day?

How many ml for a 14-day supply?

8 Your patient requires loperamide 16mg per day in two divided doses. You have 2mg tablets.

How many tablets per dose?

How many tablets per day?

How many tablets for a 14 day supply?

9 Your patient requires metoclopramide 10mg three times daily. You have 1mg per ml oral solution.

How many ml per dose?

How many ml per day?

How many ml for a 5-day supply?

10 Your patient requires prochlorperazine 20mg followed by a further 10mg after two hours. You have 5mg tablets.

How many tablets for the one-day course?

Multiple choice questions

Try answering these multiple choice questions to test what you have learned from reading this chapter. You can check your answers on page 155.

1 Cannabis falls into which class of the Misuse of Drugs Act 1971?

a) A
b) B
c) C
d) B and C

2 ← In which schedule of the Misuse of Drugs Regulations of 2001 would you find amphetamine?

a) Schedule 1
b) Schedule 2
c) Schedule 3
d) Schedule 4

3 Substance misuse is found in

a) Mainly the lower classes
b) The middle class
c) People under the age of 50
d) A wide range of age, cultural and socioeconomic backgrounds

4 The Medicines Act of 1968 governs

a) Production
b) Supply
c) Categorization
d) All of the above

5 Vitamin supplements are given in the treatment of

a) Alcohol-use disorders
b) Opiate addiction
c) Smoking cessation
d) Drug overdose

6 The Health and Social Care Information Centre gathers information about drug misuse from

a) Hospitals
b) Crime surveys
c) Support groups
d) All of the above

7 Methadone is given in the management of

a) Opioid misuse
b) Opioid intoxication
c) Opioid withdrawal
d) Opioid replacement

8 Muscle cramps in opiate withdrawal can be treated by giving

a) Methadone
b) Mebeverine

→

c) Prochlorperazine

d) Chlordiazepoxide

9　Methadone should be given

a) Twice daily

b) Once daily

c) Once daily and supervised

d) By IV injection

10　*Delirium tremens* is seen during withdrawal from

a) Alcohol

b) Opiates

c) Smoking

d) All of the above

Case study

Jim is a 24-year-old opiate addict who has met a girl and wants to get married. He wants to 'get clean' and has attended the drug and alcohol clinic with a view to starting methadone treatment. Establish the points the nurse should consider when assisting in his treatment and the management of his withdrawal from opiates.

Recommended websites

British National Formulary (BNF): www.bnf.org

http://knowthescore.info/

http://www.talktofrank.com/

Recommended further reading

Department of Health (2007) *Drug Misuse and Dependence: UK Guidelines on Clinical Management*. London: Department of Health. Available at http://www.nta.nhs.uk/uploads/clinical_guidelines_2007.pdf (accessed 25 February 2016).

Health and Social Care Information Centre (2014) *Statistics on Drug Misuse: England 2014*. Available at: http://www.hscic.gov.uk/catalogue/PUB15943/drug-misu-eng-2014-rep.pdf (accessed 25 February 2016).

Home Office (2014) *Drug Misuse: Findings from our 2013/2014 Crime Survey For England & Wales*. London: Home Office. Available at: https://www.gov.uk/ government/uploads/system/uploads/attachment_data/file/335989/drug_misuse_201314.pdf (accessed 2 March 2016).

National Institute for Health and Care Excellence (NICE) (2008) *Stop Smoking Services. PH10*. London: NICE. Available at: https://www.nice.org.uk/guidance/ph10 (accessed 25 February 2016).

National Institute for Health and Care Excellence (NICE) (2010) *Alcohol Use Disorders: Diagnosis and Management of Physical Complications. CG100*. London: NICE. Available at: http://www.nice.org.uk/guidance/cg100 (accessed 25 February 2016).

National Institute for Health and Care Excellence (NICE) (2011) *Alcohol-Use Disorders: Diagnosis, Assessment and Management of Harmful Drinking and Alcohol Dependence. CG115*. London: NICE. Available at: https://www.nice.org.uk/guidance/cg115 (accessed 25 February 2016).

The Crown Office (1968) *The Medicines Act 1968*. Available at: http://www.legislation.gov.uk/ukpga/1968/67/part/III (accessed 25 February 2016).

The Crown Office (1971) *The Misuse of Drugs Act 1971*. Available at: http://www.legislation.gov.uk/ukpga/1971/38/contents (accessed 25 February 2016).

The Crown Office (1988) *The Road Traffic Act 1988*. Available at: http://www.legislation.gov.uk/ukpga/1988/52/contents (accessed 25 February 2016).

The Crown Office (2001) *The Misuse of Drugs Regulations 2001*. Available at: http://www.legislation.gov.uk/uksi/2001/3998/contents/made (accessed 25 February 2016).

World Health Organization (WHO) (2016). *International Statistical Classification of Diseases and Related Health Problems 10th Revision (ICD–10) - WHO Version for 2016*. Available at: http://apps.who.int/classifications/icd10/browse/2016/en (accessed 19 February 2016).

Mental health medication in children and adolescents

12

Chapter contents

Learning objectives
Introduction
Presentation of the conditions
Physiological considerations in children and adolescents
Legal frameworks, consent and capacity
Licensing and dosing
Parental involvement

Key learning points
Multiple choice questions
Case study
Recommended websites
Recommended further reading

Learning objectives

After reading this chapter you will have gained knowledge around:

- The physiological factors to consider when using medication in children and adolescents.
- The legal aspects of medication administration in children and adolescents.
- The impact of cognitive and emotional factors.
- The role of the parent or guardian in the management of care.

Introduction

Children and adolescents are not immune from mental health disorders. They may present in a different manner or with a differing range of symptoms than adults presenting with the same condition. Careful assessment and diagnosis is required and management of the child or adolescent with a mental health disorder should be done in specialist care circumstances by healthcare professionals specially trained in the discipline. It is important that we consider special circumstances that need to be taken into account in the diagnosis, management and pharmacological treatment of this age group. It is also important that we consider the scale of the problem. A report prepared by the UK charity Young Minds (2014) outlined the following points.

- One in ten children and young people aged 5–16 suffer from a diagnosable mental health disorder – that is around three children in every class
- Between 1 in every 12 and 1 in 15 children and young people deliberately self-harm.
- There has been a big increase in the number of young people being admitted to hospital because of self-harm. Over the past 10 years this figure has increased by 68 per cent.
- More than half of all adults with mental health problems were diagnosed in childhood. Less than half were treated appropriately at the time.

- Nearly 80,000 children and young people suffer from severe depression.
- Over 8,000 children aged under 10 years old suffer from severe depression.
- 72 per cent of children in care have behavioural or emotional problems – these are some of the most vulnerable people in our society.
- 95 per cent of imprisoned young offenders have a mental health disorder. Many of them are struggling with more than one disorder.
- The number of young people aged 15–16 with depression nearly doubled between the 1980s and the 2000s.
- The proportion of young people aged 15–16 with a conduct disorder more than doubled between 1974 and 1999.

Presentation of the conditions

We have to remember that for children and adolescents, presentation of their condition requires us to conduct assessments looking at the four areas outlined in Figure 12.1.

Some of the causes or triggers for mental health disorders are similar or the same as those seen in the adult population in that they can be grouped as biological, psychological, social and environmental. But some of the triggers and some of the behavioural changes to look out for are quite specific and could be missed or misinterpreted as normal 'teenage angst' or even as bad behaviour (Table 12.1).

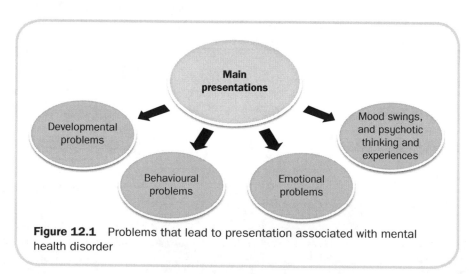

Figure 12.1 Problems that lead to presentation associated with mental health disorder

Table 12.1   Child- and adolescent-specific triggers and their related behaviours

Child- and adolescent-specific triggers/causes	Child- and adolescent-specific behaviour
Change of school	School avoidance and truancy
Exam stress	Regression in skills and poor performance
Being a child carer	Running away from home
Being in care	Separation anxiety

This list is not exhaustive but suggestive of some child- and adolescent-specific issues. Children and adolescents can suffer from a range of mental health conditions in most of the categories covered in other chapters of this book. For example:

- anxiety;
- depression;
- bipolar disorder;
- psychosis;
- eating disorders.

And some conditions that are not covered in the remit of the other chapters that may affect mental health and lead to or contribute to one of the conditions above include:

- attention–deficit hyperactivity disorder;
- attachment disorder;
- autism spectrum disorders;
- learning disability.

If we need to employ management interventions, be they psychological or pharmacological, we need to explore the physiological differences in children and we need to be aware of specific guidelines and frameworks that exist for us to practice within with regard to this patient group.

Physiological considerations in children and adolescents

Children cannot just be viewed as small adults when it comes to medication. They respond differently to drugs for many reasons, most of which can be related to pharmacokinetics, the way their body handles a drug, with respect to absorption, distribution, metabolism and excretion of drugs. Detailed explanations of these processes are not contained within this book so further reading is suggested in the form of Barber & Robertson (2015) *Essentials of Pharmacology for Nurses (3rd edition)*. A summary of the main considerations in children is presented in Box 12.1 (Barber and Robertson 2015). Let us explore each of these processes in a little more detail.

Absorption

This is an important consideration in drug administration with children under the age of 12. Delayed emptying of stomach contents means that drugs taken by the oral route stay in the stomach for longer, in turn delaying the absorption of drugs from the small intestine and beyond. Children have a longer gastrointestinal transit time, meaning that drugs and their metabolites contained in the gut stay in contact with their absorbing sites for longer. Also, it must be remembered that some young, and not so young, children have trouble swallowing tablets and often we have to be prepared to supply liquid medicines as oppose to solid dose medicines where appropriate.

Distribution

Plasma protein levels in the circulation of the child are at their lowest just after birth, especially in babies born before term. This means that the availability of proteins for drug binding is limited compared with that of an adult. This can be a problem in drugs that are highly bound to plasma proteins as a higher active dose can be seen if the dose given was an adult one. Highly plasma protein bound drugs are given in lower doses than in adults.

Box 12.1 Pharmacokinetic features in children and adolescents

Absorption (children and adolescents)	Distribution (children under 6)
■ Delayed gastric emptying ■ Slower gastrointestinal transit (longer contact) ■ Thinner skin ■ Use of rectal administration	■ Plasma protein levels lower immediately after birth, especially in premature babies ■ Presence of bilirubin can affect binding to plasma proteins ■ More body water for drug distribution
Metabolism (children under 3 months)	**Excretion (children under 6 months)**
■ Liver maturity happens quickly after birth in term babies, usually by four weeks ■ Conjugation of bilirubin occurs ■ Increased clearance after four weeks due to relative liver mass and hepatic blood flow being higher	■ Glomerular filtration is 40 per cent of adult level at birth ■ Tubular secretion processes poorly developed ■ Renal maturity slower than liver, reaching full maturity only after six months in the term infant

Metabolism

Children metabolize drugs in a different manner and at a different rate to their adult counterparts. This can lead to higher levels of an active drug being present for longer and produces a risk of toxicity. The liver takes time to mature over the first few weeks and months of life and as the liver contains the enzymes necessary for drug metabolism the immature liver cell is an important consideration in drug prescribing. It is important to remember that as a proportion of body size, the mass of the liver is larger in children than it is in adults.

Excretion

Children's kidneys are immature at birth and cannot efficiently process drug molecules. This leads to delays in excreting drug molecules that can continue to circulate for longer, again with a risk of toxicity. Renal maturity is important when prescribing for young children.

All of these effects combined result in the need for lower doses of medicines than adults, not simply because children are smaller, but due to the immaturity of many organ systems. Doses of drugs can be increased at 6 months in line with body mass calculations or national or local guidelines (the BNF for Children [BNFC] is an important source of dose information) and slowly raised to adult doses for many drugs by the age of 12, when organ maturity is achieved. From the age of 12 a child is considered pharmacologically to be able to take adult doses of medication due to a mature physiological state.

Age and physiology are not the only factors we have to consider when prescribing to a child under 12 or indeed to an adolescent with a mental health disorder. We also need to consider legal and ethical issues.

Legal frameworks, consent and capacity

With regard to children and adolescents, it is legal for healthcare professionals involved in the care of a minor to provide advice and treatment without parental consent. This can only be done providing certain criteria are met. These criteria, known as the Fraser Guidelines (sometimes called Gillick Competencies) require the professional to be satisfied that:

■ the young person will understand the professional's advice;
■ the young person cannot be persuaded to inform their parents;

- the young person is likely to begin, or to continue having, sexual intercourse with or without contraceptive treatment;
- unless the young person receives contraceptive treatment, their physical or mental health, or both, are likely to suffer;
- the young person's best interests require them to receive contraceptive advice or treatment with or without parental consent.

(Gillick v West Norfolk & Wisbech Area Health Authority [1985])

Although these criteria specifically refer to contraception, which is the court case and ruling Lord Fraser based these guidelines on, the principles are deemed to apply to other medical treatments. Although the judgement in the House of Lords that produced these criteria referred specifically to doctors, it is considered to apply to other health professionals, including nurses.

Lord Fraser specifically stated that: '. . . it is not enough that she should understand the nature of the advice which is being given: she must also have a sufficient maturity to understand what is involved'. Lord Fraser went on to give his comments more generally on parents' versus children's rights: '...parental right yields to the child's right to make his own decisions when he reaches a sufficient understanding and intelligence to be capable of making up his own mind on the matter requiring decision' (Gillick v West Norfolk & Wisbech Area Health Authority [1985]).

If a person under the age of 18 refuses to consent to treatment, it is possible in some cases for their parents or the courts to overrule their decision. However, this right can be exercised only on the basis that the welfare of the young person is paramount and they have not satisfied all of the criteria of Fraser guidance. However, it should be remembered that a child still has their right to their own self-determination and it is important to listen to the wishes of a child and give them due consideration at all times. If a decision has to be overruled this will be done by the Court of Protection, which oversees the operation and implementation of the Mental Capacity Act 2005.

Fraser Guidelines can and should be considered hand in hand with the capacity to consent that is assessed under the Mental Capacity Act 2005 that we looked at in Chapter 2, but the assessment of capacity to consent will be made using Fraser guidelines in a child. As a general rule of thumb children who are over the age of 16 are presumed to have the capacity to give consent, whereas children who are under the age of 16 are presumed to lack the capacity to give consent unless they can demonstrate that they do have the capacity after completing an assessment using the Fraser Guidelines.

In a child or adolescent with a mental health disorder capacity may already be impaired and an assessment should always take place. This falls, as you will remember from Chapter 2, under the Mental Capacity Act 2005.

Licensing and dosing

As we have alluded to above there are important considerations from a pharmacological point of view around drug doses in children. We must also be aware of the implications of licensing and drug choice and use in the child and adolescent population.

Drugs used in children and adolescents have never undergone clinical trials or testing in a child population due to the ethical implications of performing drug trials on children who may lack the capacity to consent to the trial. It is therefore commonly acknowledged that drugs given to children are used in an unlicensed or off-licence manner. Each drug has a product licence for the UK and may be prescribed but in general it is not specifically licensed for use in children or adolescents. This practice of prescribing medications for children, coupled with good monitoring and review, means that we frequently do not consider licensing status when medications are given to children. Many medications used in mental health, however, do not have guideline doses or prescribing information for children when we look them up in the BNF. Specific guidance therefore on prescribing in children and adolescents must be taken from elsewhere when we consider these medications.

The General Medical Council gives doctors very specific guidelines when prescribing unlicensed medicines to patients. They outline the areas where unlicensed prescribing is permissible and appropriate. These include:

- where no suitable licensed medication meets the patient's needs (this can include prescribing for children);
- the patient needs an unlicensed medication when the licensed alternative is not available (this may be due to supply issues or may cover specially prepared liquid formulations).

In the following five short sections we will consider some of the main medications that are used in mental health nursing for children and adolescents. It is important that you gain a working familiarity with these medications used in practice. You should be able to use the BNF to look up the medicines and to ascertain any effects and side-effects your patients may experience. You should also be able to use Appendix One of the BNF to check for interactions that these medications may have with other medications your patient may be taking at the same time.

Medications used in anxiety

There is very little guidance or information for the use of the traditional medicines for anxiety that we discussed in Chapter 6. The BNF gives only adult doses and does not specify how much can be given to children for the indication of the relief of anxiety. Anxiety is a subsection of mental health disorders in the chapter on the nervous system in the BNF, but when we look at the BNFC we see that anxiety is not present. This gives no prescribing information or dosing to go on. This is not because children and adolescents do not experience anxiety but rather that management of anxiety by medication is not the first-line treatment or highly recommended. The first-line of anxiety management in children and adolescents is usually a talking therapy such as CBT. If this is not successful or sufficient then a medical practitioner experienced in the management of mental health disorders in children (namely a psychiatrist) may prescribe an

SSRI (normally used in depression) for the child. They are not recommended for use in the under-18s due to the increased risk of side-effects or adverse effects but may be considered if the anxiety is severe enough. The prescription in this case will only be considered if the benefits outweigh the risks and talking therapy continues. Fluoxetine is usually the first choice of SSRI.

Medication used in depression

The SSRIs are the drug of choice in the child or adolescent with depression who has been unresponsive to talking therapies. Again as above, it should be used in conjunction with the talking therapy and initiated and monitored under specialist supervision by a psychiatrist. NICE did publish a clinical guideline (CG28) around management of depression in children and young people but this is dated 2005 and is in need of review. However, NICE do have a quality statement from 2013 (QS48) that is aimed at improving care in this area of practice. It provides guidance around process and refers to the recommendations in CG28 (NICE 2005) for treatment options, outlining a stepped-care model, which can be seen in Box 12.2.

These guidelines are still in current use and all the antidepressant medications listed in the table are found, with prescribing guidance in the BNFC; however, citalopram still is not licensed for use in children according to BNFC (2015–2016).

Medication used in bipolar affective disorder

Lithium, the mainstay of medication management in bipolar disorder in adults can also be used in children and adolescents if a definitive diagnosis of the disorder has been made by a medical practitioner experienced in the management of mental health disorders in children (namely a psychiatrist). The use of lithium in this age group is restricted in the BNFC to ages 12–17 years. This is partly because it is unlikely that a firm diagnosis could be made under 12 years of age, but also because a drug such as lithium, which has a narrow therapeutic window as we discussed in Chapter 10, would be less safe to give under the age of 12 when renal and hepatic maturity had not reached its maximum.

Box 12.2   Stepped care approach to depression

Focus	Action
Detection	Risk profiling
Recognition	Identification in presenting children or young people
Mild depression	Watchful waiting Non-directive supportive therapy/group CBT/ guided self-help
Moderate to severe depression	Brief psychological therapy with or without fluoxetine
Depression unresponsive to treatment/ recurrent depression/psychotic depression	Intensive psychological therapy with or without fluoxetine, sertraline, citalopram, augmentation with an antipsychotic

Medications used in psychosis

There is good guidance issued by NICE on the use of pharmacological management of psychosis and schizophrenia in children and young people (CG155, NICE 2013). As a disorder that is primarily diagnosed in the adolescent years, commencement of medication is entirely appropriate at the time diagnosis is established. Again diagnosis should be made by a medical practitioner experienced in the management of mental health disorders in children (namely a psychiatrist).

The guidance from NICE states that the choice of antipsychotic medication should be made by the parents or carers of younger children, or jointly with the young person and their parents or carers, and the healthcare professional involved. The healthcare professional should provide age-appropriate information to allow an informed choice. Most of the antipsychotics we discussed in Chapter 8 can be prescribed in the 12–17 or 15–17 age groups, but some drugs, mostly from the typical category, can be prescribed to even younger children. Precautions and preliminary assessment before commencement should be the same as in adults, which we looked at in Chapter 8.

There is more evidence around the use of, and the guidelines supporting, some antipsychotics over others. The NICE technology appraisal guideline (TA213, 2011) looks at the specific use of aripiprazole for the treatment of schizophrenia in people aged 15 to 17 years. It looks at relative risks of antipsychotics and considers the evidence. It states that adolescents with the disorder are more likely to be treated on low doses of antipsychotics and subject to closer monitoring than their adult counterparts. Its recommendations were that aripiprazole is to be considered in people aged 15–17 years who are intolerant to risperidone or for whom risperidone is contraindicated.

Medications used in eating disorders

As we will see in Chapter 13 there is a very small evidence base around the effectiveness of pharmacological interventions in the main eating disorder of anorexia nervosa. Medications that can be used are often aimed at treating the comorbid conditions that often accompany it such as depression and anxiety. Like in adults, medication should not be used as the sole treatment for anorexia nervosa.

There are other special considerations in children and adolescents with anorexia nervosa. Family interventions are recommended but along with family therapy, children and adolescents should be offered individual appointments with their healthcare professional. Involvement of siblings should be evaluated as part of family therapy where there is a risk of the sibling developing the disorder. Inpatient assessment should only be considered after balancing the health and welfare needs of the child against their educational and social needs. In the case of interventions where feeding against the will of the patient is considered this should only be done in the context of the Mental Health Act 1983 and the Children Act 1989.

In bulimia nervosa some evidence exists to show benefit in the prescribing of SSRIs. The effective dose of fluoxetine (the first-line SSRI of choice) is higher than that used in depression. This should be given in combination with psychological therapies that should follow the special considerations outlined under anorexia nervosa, but specific targeted CBT should also be considered. There is also further guidance from NICE (CG9, 2004).

Parental involvement

Parental involvement should be sought and encouraged where it is appropriate to do so. In a child under the age of 16 who is not deemed to have capacity to consent by Fraser Guidelines, the parent has the legal responsibility to give or withhold consent on their behalf. If a parent chooses to withhold consent that is deemed necessary by the healthcare professional then a court can overrule this. If a decision has to be overruled this will be done by the Court of Protection, which oversees the operation and implementation of the Mental Capacity Act 2005.

In the event of two people with parental responsibility disagreeing about whether or not consent to proceed should be given, the healthcare professionals involved in the care have the legal right to accept the decision of consent of one parent and carry out the intervention. There is provision in law where if a person who holds parental responsibility is not available to give consent and the treatment or intervention is deemed to be necessary to avoid undue extreme risk, then care can proceed in the absence of consent.

It is important also to remember that the person with legal parental responsibility does not need to be the child's biological parent. The person holding the power to make the decisions could be:

- the parent, be that the mother or father;
- a legally appointed guardian;
- someone who holds a residency order concerning the child in question;
- the local authority designated to care for the child or their representative;
- the local authority or a designated person with an emergency protection order for the child in question.

These are outlined in more detail in the Children Act 1989.

It is important to remember that children and adolescents differ in the way their conditions should be managed and I hope this chapter has helped further your understanding of the differences in treatment from a legal and pharmacological perspective.

Key learning points

Physiological considerations

▶ Pharmacokinetic considerations around the areas of drug absorption, distribution, metabolism and excretion need to be considered before prescribing takes place.
▶ Age-appropriate prescribing should be carried out using dosing information and guidance found in the BNFC.

$\longrightarrow$

Legal aspects

▶ Capacity and consent should be conducted around the Mental Capacity Act 2005 and following Fraser Guidelines.

Licensing and dosing

▶ Many drugs used in the child and adolescent age group do not have licensing for use.
▶ Drugs can be prescribed off-licence or can be prescribed even if they are to be used in an unlicensed form.
▶ Suitable licensed alternatives should always be considered.

Parental role

▶ Parental responsibility should be ascertained and parental involvement encouraged where appropriate to do so.
▶ People who can hold parental responsibility are outlined in the Children Act 1989.

Multiple choice questions

Try answering these multiple choice questions to test what you have learned from reading this chapter. You can check your answers on page 155.

1 **How can capacity to consent be assessed in a child?**

a) Mental Health Act
b) Human Rights Act
c) Fraser Guidelines
d) Using the parent to judge

2 **What other piece of legislation should be considered when asking for consent in a child or adolescent?**

a) Mental Health Act
b) Human Rights Act
c) The Children's Act
d) Mental Capacity Act

3 **Parental involvement in decision making should be**

a) Encouraged
b) Avoided
c) Only sought as a last resort
d) Unnecessary

4 **What is the number of the NICE clinical guideline around eating disorder management?**

a) CG9

→

b) CG28

c) CG115

d) CG155

5 What is the first-line SSRI of choice in depression in children and young people?

a) Citalopram

b) Sertraline

c) Fluoxetine

d) Paroxetine

6 Aripiprazole is recommended for

a) Children with a diagnosis of schizophrenia

b) Children with a diagnosis of schizophrenia aged 15–17 as first line

c) Children with a diagnosis of schizophrenia aged 15–17 if they ask for it

d) Children with a diagnosis of schizophrenia aged 15–17 if they are intolerant to risperidone

7 Anxiety management in children should consist of what first-line treatment?

a) Talking therapy

b) Benzodiazepines

c) Hypnotics

d) Buspirone

8 Plasma protein binding affects which aspect of pharmacodynamics?

a) Absorption

b) Distribution

c) Metabolism

d) Excretion

9 Best prescribing guidelines for children and adolescents can be found in

a) The BNF

b) The BNFC

c) From your peers

d) From the child you are prescribing for

10 What can be looked up in Appendix One of the BNF?

a) Drug doses

b) Drug names

c) Drug interactions

d) Drug effects

Case study

Jack Smith is a 15-year-old schoolboy suffering from depression and anxiety. He is a second child and works very hard at school to try to get good results as he wants to go to university like his brother who is studying law at Cambridge. Exams are looming and he cannot sleep or concentrate. He is worrying constantly that he will not succeed and is pessimistic about his chances. He cannot remember the last time he enjoyed anything and says he will kill himself if he fails. His parents are very supportive and do not pressure Jack at all.

What are the treatment options for a teenager with depression and how else may the nurse support Jack?

Recommended websites

British National Formulary (BNF) and British National Formulary for Children (BNFC) both at: www.bnf.org
EMC medicines compendium: www.medicines.org.uk
Young Minds website: www.youngminds.org.uk

Recommended further reading

Barber, P. and Robertson, D. (2015) *Essentials of Pharmacology for Nurses, 3rd edn*. Maidenhead: Open University Press. British and Irish Legal Information Institute (BAILII) (1985) *Gillick v West Norfolk & Wisbech Area Health Authority* [1985] UKHL 7.

National Institute for Health and Care Excellence (NICE) (2004) *Eating Disorders in Over 8s: Management. CG9*. London: NICE. Available at: https://www.nice.org.uk/guidance/cg9 (accessed 25 February 2016).

National Institute for Health and Care Excellence (NICE) (2005) *Depression in Children and Young People: Identification and Management. CG28*. London: NICE. Available at: https://www.nice.org.uk/guidance/cg28 (accessed 25 February 2016).

National Institute for Health and Care Excellence (NICE) (2011) *Aripiprazole for the Treatment of Schizophrenia in People Aged 15 to 17 Years. TA213*. London: NICE. Available at: https://www.nice.org.uk/guidance/ta213 (accessed 25 February 2016).

National Institute for Health and Care Excellence (NICE) (2013) *Psychosis and Schizophrenia in Children and Young People: Recognition and Management. CG155*. London: NICE. Available at: https://www.nice.org.uk/guidance/cg155 (accessed 25 February 2016).

National Institute for Health and Care Excellence (NICE) (2013) *Depression in Children and Young People. QS48*. London: NICE. Available at: https://www.nice.org.uk/guidance/qs48 (accessed 25 February 2016).

National Institute for Health and Care Excellence (NICE) (2015) *Bipolar Disorder, Psychosis and Schizophrenia in Children and Young People. QS102*. London: NICE. Available at: https://www.nice.org.uk/guidance/qs102 (accessed 25 February 2016).

The Crown Office (1983) *Mental Health Act 1983*. Available at: http://www.legislation.gov.uk/ukpga/1983/20/contents (accessed 25 February 2016).

The Crown Office (1989) *Children Act 1989*. Available at: http://www.legislation.gov.uk/ukpga/1989/41/contents(accessed 25 February 2016).

The Crown Office (2005) *Mental Capacity Act 2005*. Available at: http://www.legislation.gov.uk/ukpga/2005/9/contents (accessed 2 February 2016).

The Crown Office (2007) *Mental Health Act 2007*. Available at: http://www.legislation.gov.uk/ukpga/2007/12/contents (accessed 25 February 2016).

Young Minds (2014) *What's the Problem*. London: Young Minds. Available at: http://www.youngminds.org.uk/about/whats_the_problem (accessed 25 February 2016).

Eating disorders

13

Chapter contents

Learning objectives

After reading this chapter you will have gained knowledge around:

- The incidence and classification of eating disorders as a mental health issue.
- The typical interventions used in the management of eating disorders.
- The pharmacodynamic actions of drugs used in the management of eating disorders.

Introduction

Eating disorders have been around for a very long time and disturbances in what are deemed to be 'normal' eating patterns can often be seen in many people in many areas of our society. The actual diagnosis of eating disorders as mental health issues has a more rigid approach that we will look at. You may find, however, that some people will include all of the following in their idea of what constitutes a deviation from normal eating patterns:

- the role of eating in child development (socialization; celebration);
- temporary changes in eating (illness; routines; stress; control; depression);
- the role of media, fashion and friends as drivers for weight management;
- food continuum (fussy or faddy; restricted eating; food refusal);
- anorexia nervosa;
- bulimia nervosa.

Only the last two can be considered true eating disorders and these are what we will focus this chapter on.

The classifications of eating disorder

Anorexia nervosa

This is a condition in which there is deliberate weight loss. It is most common in adolescent girls and young women but is also seen in males in these age groups. It is also seen in older age groups right up to pre-menopausal women. There is no recognized underlying cause but it is thought that there are biological and cultural drivers underlying the condition. The associated under-nutrition causes endocrine and metabolic changes that can in turn result in disturbances in bodily function. A diagnosis can be made when the following criteria are met.

- The patient's body weight is consistently more than 15 per cent below what might be expected.
- Body mass index is 17.5 or less.
- The weight loss is self-induced.
- There is distorted body image.

- There is a disruption of the hypothalamic–pituitary–gonadal axis with amenorrhoea (an abnormal absence of menstruation) in women and loss of sexual interest and potency in men.
- If onset is prepubertal there may be an associated delay in pubertal development, or it may fail to occur.

Much has been made in the media and by medical professionals who work in this area about the role of models and the culture in the fashion media for an extreme thin frame, the so called 'size 0' as a driver for or an underlying cause of anorexia or anorexic behaviour. There is some aspect of truth in this as patients who are in talking therapies will discuss the 'pressures' to be thin and to conform to what is seen as a societal norm or a desired body shape. Very often this can be through peer pressure as much as media and societal pressure to achieve a target weight that the person suffering from anorexia may have set themselves.

Bulimia nervosa

This is characterized by bouts of over-eating. These are followed by behaviour designed to offset the effects of the excessive calorie intake. It is sometimes described as bingeing and purging. This may take the form of self-induced vomiting, purgative abuse, and prolonged periods of starvation. Drugs that might alter weight may also be abused such as thyroid hormones, appetite suppressants or diuretics. It is thought that the underlying cause is a morbid fear of fatness that leads the patient to adopt a strict upper weight level that they will then attempt to stay below at all cost. The age groups involved are similar to those seen with anorexia nervosa and it is not uncommon for patients with bulimia to have had a previous diagnosis of anorexia. Excessive vomiting or purgative use can result in electrolyte imbalance and this may constitute the presenting feature as this leads to systemic unwellness.

As we can see the predominance of this is in the adolescent age group and we must be mindful of the legal and professional issues we discussed around capacity and consent in this age group in Chapter 12.

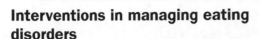

Interventions in managing eating disorders

The management of anorexia nervosa is with the use of talking therapies as can be seen from guidance issued by NICE (CG9, 2004). The aim is risk reduction and this is done by encouraging healthy eating and weight gain. There is only a very limited place for the use of medication and that is in the management of the symptoms associated with the disease rather than in treatment of the condition itself. Even then it is important to point out that most of the physical symptoms of the disease will settle if there is adequate weight gain.

In the case of bulimia nervosa there is a place for the use of high doses of SSRIs, usually fluoxetine at a dose of 60mg or 80mg daily. Apart from this the mainstay of treatment is again talking therapies.

Pharmacology of medication used in management of eating disorders

As there are so few pharmacological interventions seen in eating disorders we have very little pharmacology to discuss. The SSRIs, namely fluoxetine, and the mechanism of action around serotonin levels and receptor activation have been discussed in Chapter 7 on depression.

However, you will see that the dose used in bulimia nervosa is considerably higher than the dose that we use in depressive disorders. There is a pharmacological reason for this. It had been assumed that using SSRIs had its primary effect in eating disorders by treating underlying and/or comorbid depression, which would allow the patient to resume a normal eating habit and pattern, and indeed this may in part be true. But at higher doses of fluoxetine, such as we see used here, there are other effects of the medication that are not seen, or are only partly seen, at the lower therapeutic doses used in depression. They appear to help with regulation of the binge–purge cycle that is typical of bulimia nervosa and have a stabilizing effect on emotions. At high doses they also help to regulate hunger signals, which may be the trigger for binge eating.

As with other areas of medicines management, it is important that you gain a working familiarity with these medications used in practice. You should be able to use the BNF to look up the medicines and to ascertain any effects and side-effects your patients may experience. You should also be able to use Appendix One of the BNF to check for interactions that these medications may have with other medications your patient may be taking at the same time.

Key learning points

Classifications of eating disorders

► There are many deviations from what is considered normal eating but a true eating disorder shows the signs and symptoms discussed under anorexia nervosa and bulimia nervosa.

Physiology and pharmacology

► The causes of eating disorders are thought to mainly be biopsychosocial.
► Pharmacological intervention in the management of eating disorders is limited.
► Talking therapies and counselling form the mainstay of intervention.

Multiple choice questions

Try answering these multiple choice questions to test what you have learned from reading this chapter. You can check your answers on page 156.

1 Anorexia nervosa can be diagnosed with a body mass index of ____ or less

a) 20
b) 17.5
c) 15
d) 12.5

2 What is the characteristic cycle in bulimia nervosa?

a) Binge/purge
b) Binge/starve
c) Starve/binge
d) Starve/purge

3 What is the main intervention in eating disorders?

a) Antipsychotics
b) SSRIs
c) Talking therapy
d) All of the above

4 Which SSRI is used in bulimia nervosa?

a) Paroxetine
b) Citalopram
c) Sertraline
d) Fluoxetine

5 What is the main age group for diagnosis of an eating disorder?

a) Under 12
b) 12–18
c) 18–25
d) Over 25

6 What is the number of the NICE clinical guideline addressing eating disorders?

a) CG9
b) CG90
c) CG99
d) CG115

7 What signals can SSRIs help to regulate in bulimia nervosa?

a) Fullness
b) Nausea
c) Hunger
d) Pain

$\longrightarrow$

8 What is the main aim of NICE clinical guidelines around eating disorders?

a) Weight gain
b) Weight stabilization
c) Medication
d) Risk reduction

9 Media influence has been seen as a trigger in eating disorders as girls, particularly, aim for what size?

a) Size 0
b) Size 6
c) Size 8
d) Size 10

10 Legal capacity to consent to treatment for eating disorders

a) Should be considered using the Mental Health Act
b) Should be considered using the Mental Capacity Act
c) Should be considered using the Fraser Guidelines
d) All of the above

Case study

Emily Peters is a 22-year-old girl who lives at home with her parents. She admits to being obsessed with how she looks and cannot bear the thought of gaining weight. These ideas completely absorb her and everything she does and thinks about are around keeping thin. She tries to eat normally around her parents but ensures she can use the bathroom after meals so she can vomit. She regularly takes laxatives. She does not eat at all outside the home. She is now convinced she is fat and has stopped eating completely. Her current body mass index is 13. Outline the treatment options for Emily.

Recommended websites

Beating Eating Disorders: http://www.b-eat.co.uk/
British National Formulary (BNF) and British National Formulary for Children (BNFC): www.bnf.org
EMC medicines compendium: www.medicines.org.uk
Young Minds website: www.youngminds.org.uk

Recommended further reading

National Institute for Health and Care Excellence (NICE) (2004) *Eating Disorders in Over 8s: Management.* CG9. Available at: https://www.nice.org.uk/guidance/cg9 (accessed 25 February 2016).

Conclusion

It is, without doubt, a simple fact that to be a safe practitioner with regard to medicines management, the nurse must have a good, applied knowledge of pharmacology, physiology and pathology. In addition, they must be able to complete simple drug calculations and be aware of legal and practical aspects of medicines management. This book's aim was to introduce you to the underpinning theory and practical application to allow you to undertake this important part of a nurse's role.

As a nurse, the mainstay of your role is to provide and facilitate care for the patients you come into contact with. It is important that any topic area, such as pharmacology, is practically applied to your nursing practice. The information on clinical processes and case studies throughout this book has been designed to give you an insight into the importance of understanding pharmacology and to be relevant to the nursing care you provide.

Chapter summaries

Chapter 1

In this chapter we had an introduction to mental health and the disorders that can affect it. We were introduced to the ICD-10 (WHO 2016), the system of classification of disease, and this was to be referred to where appropriate throughout the rest of the book. The classifications of mental health disorder were outlined and we discussed the aims of treatment of any mental health disorder, which is to promote recovery and return the patient to a functional capacity. The prevalence of mental health disorders was investigated and related to the UK population. We also started to look at the mental health nurse and their role in current society and healthcare. This chapter sets the scene for the rest of the book.

Chapter 2

In this chapter we looked at the legislation and professional and ethical considerations with regard to people with a mental health disorder. The issue of consent was addressed along with aspects around treatment delivery if consent was refused. This is an important chapter as the mental health nurse must be familiar with the legal, professional and ethical frameworks that surround their practice.

Chapter 3

Here we looked at the concept of medicines management, what it meant and how nurses in the mental health arena should be involved, especially their function within the MDT. In this chapter we also considered the important area of drug calculation, with examples.

Chapter 4

This is where we take a deeper look at relationships, roles and responsibilities regarding the patient's adherence to their medication regime and the concept of the therapeutic alliance was introduced. Patient health beliefs were considered and so were those of relatives and carers. The nurse's role in this process was examined.

Chapter 5

In Chapter 5 we looked at the anatomy and physiology of the brain. Structural components are outlined and functional attributes addressed where appropriate. The roles and functions of nerve cells and the synapse are explained, as well as the concept of monoamines and neurotransmission. This helps to build up a picture of normal physiological structure and function. It is from this basis that we can then explore pathophysiology and the basis of pharmacological interventions in later chapters.

Chapter 6

This is the first of the chapters that deals with mental health disorders themselves. Individuals with anxiety disorders make up a significant proportion of patients presenting to mental health services and anxiety itself and related disorders are explored within this chapter. We then go on to cover the range and actions of common medications used in the management of these disorders while acknowledging the place of talking therapies and non-pharmacological management.

Chapter 7

This chapter deals with depressive disorders. Again these conditions contribute significantly to the workload of the mental health nurse and are worthy of attention. We investigate the reasons for depressive illness and then go on to look at the range and actions of common medications used in the management of these disorders while acknowledging the place of talking therapies and non-pharmacological management.

Chapter 8

Here we focus on schizophrenia and the psychotic disorders, a significant range of conditions with features of teenage onset and being lifelong in nature. Various theories around the development and aetiology are discussed with the most common hypotheses being explored in detail. We then looked at the range and actions of common medications used in the management of these disorders while acknowledging the place of talking therapies and non-pharmacological management.

Chapter 9

This chapter addresses the dementias, and although many forms of dementia are outlined the focus of the chapter is on the most common and prevalent form of dementia, that of Alzheimer's disease. We look at the guidance around diagnosis, treatment and management of the disease along with identifying factors. Pharmacological treatment is considered in the areas of cognitive decline and of symptom management.

Chapter 10

Here we look at bipolar affective disorder and other mania-related conditions. We focus on lithium as it remains a major player in the pharmacological management of the condition but explore newer therapeutic interventions and management

not forgetting the role of talking therapies in each aspect of the typical patient cycle.

Chapter 11

This is where we consider the complex treatment and management of the range of conditions and cases that make up substance misuse. We look at social and environmental factors as well as triggers and issues around reporting. Pharmacological interventions discussed include those used in managing alcohol-use disorder and opiate abuse.

Chapter 12

This chapter looks at the legal, professional and pharmacological aspects that should be considered when prescribing in the child or adolescent patient presenting with a mental health disorder. Areas include pharmacokinetics and physiological considerations as well as legal issues around consent and capacity. We also look at licensing and dosing schedules that must be adhered to. Finally, we consider the role of the parent or guardian.

Chapter 13

In our final chapter we look at the management and care of the patient presenting with an eating disorder. We focus on anorexia nervosa and bulimia nervosa and acknowledge the lack of evidence around the success of pharmacological interventions and guidance on prescribing in these areas. The first line of treatment remains talking therapies. We also discussed the importance of capacity and consent.

Throughout the book we have referred to the ICD-10 classification (WHO 2016), which has been invaluable in the classifications of the mental health disorders we have been considering.

Overall I hope this book has given you the motivation and interest to want to increase your knowledge in this important area of nursing practice. There are many books, journals and websites as well as other resources you can utilize and refer to as you become more knowledgeable and develop your understanding (see the suggestions for further reading throughout the book).

I hope that this book is a helpful part of your chosen career as a mental health nurse.

Glossary

A

absorption: process by which a drug reaches the general circulation and becomes biologically available.

acetylcholine: chemical transmitter released by certain nerve endings.

adrenaline: hormone produced by the adrenal medulla to prepare the body for fight or flight.

agonist: a drug that binds to a receptor and activates a response.

antagonist: a drug that binds to a receptor but does not activate a response or blocks the receptor to the action of its endogenous agonist.

D

distribution: the distribution of drugs after absorption, to reach their target sites.

dopamine: neurotransmitter implicated in movement and mood.

E

elimination: removal of drugs and their metabolites from the body.

G

gamma-aminobutyric acid (GABA): neurotransmitter associated with a dampening effect on brain activity.

H

half-life: the time needed for the initial concentration of the drug in plasma to fall by 50 per cent.

I

incidence: the number of times a particular phenomenon is observed or the number of people known to suffer from a particular condition.

N

neologism: a newly used or adopted word, term, phrase or expression.

neuroleptics: antipsychotic drugs.

neuron: a cell structure found in the brain and central nervous system.

P

plasma protein: proteins carried in the plasma with a range of physiological functions. Target sites for drug binding.

S

serotonin: neurotransmitter implicated in alterations of mood also known as 5-hydroxytryptamine.

synapse: the physical space between two neurons.

T

therapeutic index: this is the comparison of the amount of a drug needed to bring about a therapeutic response to the amount that would cause a toxic effect.

therapeutic range: the range of plasma concentration where medicine has its best effect.

thought broadcasting: a symptom in psychosis where the sufferer believes that their thoughts can be heard by others.

thought echo: a symptom in psychosis where the sufferer hears voices that are or appear to be repeating the persons own thoughts. A form of auditory hallucination.

thought insertion: a symptom in psychosis where the sufferer believes they are thinking through the mind of another person. A form of delusional behaviour.

thought withdrawal: a symptom in psychosis where the sufferer believes their thoughts are being taken or 'stolen' from their minds.

W

waxy flexibility: term used in assessing psychosis, refers to the reduced motor response to stimuli and the tendency towards immobility of limbs or posture.

Answers

Chapter 1

Multiple choice questions

1 D
2 A
3 D
4 C
5 A
6 C
7 D
8 B
9 A
10 D

Chapter 2

Multiple choice questions

1 D
2 D
3 D
4 A
5 C
6 C
7 C
8 B
9 A
10 C

Case study

You should be reflecting around the following points:

■ Capacity – under the Mental Capacity Act 2005 the patient will have had to be assessed by a medical professional experienced in this assessment and involved in the care of the patient. After this assessment the patient may be given treatment without consent in their best interest if they have been deemed not to have the capacity to give valid consent.

■ Consent can be written, verbal or implied and must be given freely by a person deemed to have capacity to consent. Consent without information about the treatment in a form understood by the patient is not valid.

■ Ethics. It is an ethical challenge to give medication without consent and the principles of ethics should be considered:

   ■ autonomy – the patient's rights as an individual should be respected and they should be involved in the process as much as possible;

   ■ beneficence – the nurse is obliged to do what is in the patient's best interests;

   ■ non-maleficence – no intent to do harm; the patient needs the treatment;

   ■ justice – treatment under mental health care law and capacity law should be fairly applied;

   ■ veracity – the truth of the matter should be given to the patient and any relatives or carers.

■ Professional responsibility – your code of conduct asks you to behave in a way that adheres to it and upholds ethical and moral principles including the needs of the patient.

■ The law states that you must follow process and procedure in admission of this person to hospital and it would be wise to look at circumstances of admission and status at the time of treatment. Was the patient subject to any section of the Mental Health Act? If so was consent required to be sought? If so was it sought in the proper manner and incapacity deemed to be the case? If not, then was treatment administered without consent under the appropriate section of the law?

Chapter 3

Calculations

1 $4 \times 1000 = 4000$mg

2 $2.75 \times 1000 = 2750$mg

3 $0.3 \times 1000 = 300$ng

4 $475/1000 = 0.475$g

5 $800/1000 = 0.8$mg

6 $1 \times 1000 = 1000$mg

   $1000/500 \times 1 = 2$ tablets

7 $2.4 \times 1000 = 2400$mg

   $2400/600 \times 1 = 4$ tablets

8 $360/120 \times 5 = 15$ml

9 $250/62.5 \times 2 = 8$ml

10 $0.1 \times 1000 = 100$mg

   $100/50 \times 2 = 4$ml

Multiple choice questions

1 B
2 C
3 D
4 A
5 A
6 B
7 D
8 B
9 D
10 A

Case Study

Use the 'five rights' to structure your actions:

■ *The right patient*
Confirming identity with the patient verbally where they have capacity to do so and checking details with the patient identification bracelet if present. These details should be compared with the medication prescription chart to verify the *right patient* receives the medication. This is the first thing to do.

■ *The right medication*
Check the packaging for the generic name to verify that the *right medication* is given. It is important that the nurse knows what the drug is given to treat and this can be checked in the BNF. At this point you should consult the BNF and ensure the medication is appropriate for the patient in front of you.

■ *The right time*
Does the timing of the drug, that is, daily/twice daily etc. fit with the information in the BNF? Query it with the prescriber if it does not. Sometimes drugs

can be given at different times if there is a good reason.

■ *The right dose*
Check the normal dose range in the BNF; does the drug chart match? Query it with the prescriber if it does not. Sometimes drugs can be given at different doses if there is a good reason. The drug may be written up as a set dose but the nurse may have different strength tablets to supply and calculation of how many tablets is then required. Perform any calculations necessary using the basic formula method.

■ *The right route*
Is the route prescribed appropriate? Check in the BNF and check your patient can tolerate this route. Report any difficulties in the patient taking the medication to the prescriber.

Chapter 4

Calculations

1 $200/50 \times 1 = 4$ tablets per dose

   $4 \times 2 = 8$ tablets per day

2 $600/300 \times 1 = 2$ tablets per dose

   $2 \times 4 = 8$ tablets per day

3 $3g \times 1000 = 3000$mg

   $3000/500 = 6$ tablets per day

   $6 \times 3 = 18$ tablets per day

4 $800/4 = 200$mg per dose

   $200/100 \times 1 = 2$ tablets per dose

   $2 \times 4 = 8$ tablets per day

5 $0.125g \times 1000 = 125$mg

   $375/125 \times 5 = 15$ml per dose

   $15 \times 4 = 60$ml per day

6 $1.25g \times 1000 = 1250$mg

   $1250/250 \times 2 = 10$ml per dose

   $10 \times 2 = 20$ml per day

7 $500/250 \times 5 = 10$ml for the dose

   $10 \times 10 = 100$ seconds or 1 minute 40 seconds

8 $20/2 \times 1 = 10$ml for the dose

9 $4.5/1.5 \times 1 = 3$ml for the dose

10 $80/20 \times 5 = 20$ml for the dose

Multiple choice questions

1. A
2. D
3. C
4. A
5. D
6. C
7. B
8. A
9. D
10. A

Case study

- A full discussion should take place between your patient and the doctor prescribing the medication.
- The patient should be allowed to express her feelings and opinions.
- The prescriber should outline the benefits of taking the antipsychotic medication and the risks to their mental health state if the medication is stopped.
- If appropriate, capacity to consent should be assessed and progression to changes in treatment based on the outcome of the assessment.

Chapter 5

Multiple choice questions

1. A
2. C
3. D
4. A
5. B
6. D
7. B
8. C
9. A
10. A

Chapter 6

Calculations

1. $4/2 \times 1 = 2$ tablets per dose

   $2 \times 4 = 8$ tablets per day

   $8 \times 28 = 224$ tablets for a 28-day supply

2. $40/10 \times 1 = 4$ tablets per dose

   12 hourly equals $2 \times$ per day so $4 \times 2 = 8$ per day

   $7 \times 8 = 56$ tablets for a 7-day supply

3. $15/5 \times 1 = 3$ tablets per dose

   $3 \times 2 = 6$ per day

4. $7.5/3.75 \times 1 = 2$ tablets per dose

   $28 \times 2 = 56$ tablets for a 28-day supply

5. $300/150 \times 1 = 2$ tablets per dose

   $2 \times 2 = 4$ tablets per day

   $4 \times 28 = 112$ tablets for a 28-day supply

6. $25/25 \times 1 = 1$ tablet per day $\times 7 = 7$ tablets for week 1

   $25/25 \times 1 = 1$ tablet per dose $\times 2 = 2$ tablets per day $\times 7 = 14$ tablets for week 2

   $50/25 \times 1 = 2$ tablets per day $\times 7 = 14$ tablets for week 3

   $50/25 \times 1 = 2$ tablets per dose $\times 2 = 4$ tablets per day $\times 7 = 28$ tablets for week 4

   $7 + 14 + 14 + 28 = 63$ tablets for the 28-day supply

7. $75/50 \times 5 = 7.5$ml per day

   28×7.5ml $= 210$ml for a 28-day supply

8. $10/2 \times 1 = 5$ml per day

   $5 \times 28 = 140$ml for a 28-day supply

9. $25/5 \times 1 = 5$ml per dose

   $5 \times 3 = 15$ml per day

10. $500/250 \times 1 = 2$ tablets per dose

    $3 \times 2 = 6$ tablets per day

Multiple choice questions

1. B
2. C
3. B
4. C
5. D
6. C
7. B
8. C

9 A

10 D

Case study 1, Mrs Lee

■ Mrs Lee is most likely to have GAD.

■ Talking therapy/relaxation/support groups would be very beneficial to her to help manage the day-to-day lifestyle that has contributed to her current condition.

■ Benzodiazepines at a low dose for a short time would relieve the acute symptoms of anxiety she is experiencing but care should be taken due to the propensity for them to cause addiction.

■ Beta blockers to manage symptoms may be something she would consider in the medium to long term if physical symptoms were especially problematic.

■ Review her at regular intervals to check her progress.

Case study 2, James Jackson

■ James is most likely to be suffering from PTSD related to his time in the forces and the events he has witnessed.

■ Pharmacological interventions such as SSRIs to help with the symptoms he is experiencing may be helpful as indeed may a hypnotic drug in the short term to aid his sleep.

■ Counselling and support should be offered to James and it would be good to get him in contact with people who have had similar experiences to himself through support groups and charities such as The Royal British Legion and Help for Heroes.

Chapter 7

Calculations

1 $40/20 \times 1 = 2$ tablets per day

$2 \times 28 = 56$ tablets for a 28-day supply

2 $150/50 \times 1 = 3$ tablets per dose

$28 \times 3 = 84$ tablets for a 28-day supply

3 $300/2 = 150$mg per dose

$150/75 \times 1 = 2$ tablets per dose and $2 \times 2 = 4$ tablets per day

$4 \times 28 = 112$ tablets for a 28-day supply

4 $30/15 \times 1 = 2$ tablets per day

$28 \times 2 = 56$ tablets for a 28-day supply

5 $300/3 = 100$mg per dose

$100/50 \times 1 = 2$ capsules per dose and $2 \times 3 = 6$ capsules per day

$6 \times 28 = 168$ capsules for a 28-day supply

6 $210/2 = 105$mg per dose

$105/70 \times 5 = 7.5$ml per dose $\times 2 = 15$ml per day

$15 \times 28 = 420$ml for a 28-day supply

7 $300/150 \times 1 = 2$ tablets per dose

$2 \times 2 = 4$ tablets per day

$4 \times 28 = 112$ tablets per day

8 1mg per drop and 20mg per ml = 20 drops per ml

$10/1 = 10$ drops per dose and per day

$20/10 = 2$ days to use 1ml

$2 \times 15 = 30$ days to use all 15ml

9 $4/4 \times 1 = 1$ tablet per dose and $1 \times 2 = 2$ tablets per day

$21 \times 2 = 42$ tablets for the first 3 weeks

$6/4 = 1.5$ tablets per dose $\times 2 = 3$ tablets per day

$3 \times 7 = 21$ tablets for the 4th week

$42 + 21 = 63$ tablets for the 28-day supply

10 $40/20 \times 5 = 10$ml per day

$10 \times 28 = 280$ml for a 28-day supply

Multiple choice questions

1 B

2 B

3 C

4 A

5 D

6 C

7 A

8 D

9 D

10 B

Case study

- NICE guidelines suggest SSRIs $+/-$ talking therapies.
- Start sertraline and review in 2–4 weeks for response and side-effects.
- Change drug if no effect on mood after 4 weeks.
- Monitor regularly in first 6 months.
- Possible use of a hypnotic.

Chapter 8

Calculations

1 $3/1.5 = 2$ tablets per dose

   $2 \times 3 = 6$ tablets per day

   $6 \times 28 = 168$ tablets for a 28-day supply

2 $15/5 = 3$ tablets per day

   $3 \times 28 = 84$ tablets for a 28-day supply

3 $10/2.5 = 4$ tablets per day

   $4 \times 28 = 112$ tablets for a 28-day supply

4 $300/2 = 150$mg per dose

   $150/25 = 6$ tablets per dose

   $6 \times 2 = 12$ tablets per day

   $12 \times 28 = 336$ tablets for a 28-day supply

5 $400/40 \times 1 = 10$ml per dose

   $10 \times 2 = 20$ml per day

   $20 \times 28 = 560$ml for a 28-day supply

6 $200/50 = 4$ tablets per dose

   $4 \times 2 = 8$ tablets per day

   $8 \times 28 = 224$ tablets for a 28-day supply

7 $25/25 = 1$ tablet per dose $\times 2 = 2$ tablets on day one

   $50/25 = 2$ tablets per dose $\times 2 = 4$ tablets on day two

   $100/25 = 4$ tablets per dose $\times 2 = 8$ tablets on day three

   $150/25 = 6$ tablets per dose $\times 2 = 12$ tablets per day on day four onwards

   $12 \times 25 = 300 + 8 + 4 + 2 = 314$ tablets for a 28-day supply

8 $12.5/25 \times 1 = 0.5$ml for the dose

9 $9/3 = 3$ tablets per dose

   $3 \times 28 = 84$ tablets for a 28-day supply

10 $148/37 = 4$ tablets per day

   $4 \times 28 = 112$ tablets for a 28-day supply

Multiple choice questions

1 B
2 D
3 A
4 D
5 B
6 A
7 A
8 D
9 B
10 D

Case study

- Establish her current medication-taking behaviour.
- Reinforce the benefits of adhering to a medication regime and suggest ways to help her improve her adherence.
- Set up a review in the short term to check on medication adherence and symptoms.

Chapter 9

Calculations

1 $10/2 \times 1 = 5$ml per dose

   $5 \times 28 = 140$ml for a 28-day supply

2 $5/5 = 1$ tablet per day

   $1 \times 14 = 14$ tablet for a 14-day supply

3 $12/8 = 1.5$ tablets per day

   $1.5 \times 28 = 42$ tablets for a 28-day supply

4 $10/1 \times 1 = 10$ml per day

   $10 \times 28 = 280$ml for a 28-day supply

5 $13.3/24 = 0.55$mg per hour

6 $20/10 \times 1 = 2$ml per day

   $50/2 = 25$ days

7 300/50 = 6 capsules per day

6 × 28 = 168 capsules for a 28-day supply

8 1 × 1000 = 1000micrograms

1000/500 = 2 tablets per dose

2 × 2 = 4 tablets per day

28/4 = 7 days

9 0.5mg × 1000 = 500micrograms

250/500 = 0.5 (half) a tablet per dose

0.5 × 2 = 1 tablet per day

1 × 28 = 28 tablets for a 28-day supply

10 15/7.5 = 2 tablets per day

2 × 28 = 56 tablets for a 28-day supply

Multiple choice questions

1 A
2 B
3 D
4 D
5 D
6 D
7 A
8 D
9 B
10 A

Case study

What is her current Mini-Mental State Examination score and what stage of Alzheimer's disease is she in? Remember the use of these drugs is only of proven benefit in mild to moderate disease.

■ What are her other health conditions, and is she on any other medication that may prevent her starting these drugs?
■ What is her ability to adhere to the medication regime and how much support does she have?
■ Have other non-pharmacological interventions been considered?

Chapter 10

Calculations

1 500/250 = 2 tablets per dose

2 × 3 = 6 tablets per day

2 1g × 1000 = 1000mg

1000/250 = 4 tablets per day

4 × 7 = 28 tablets for a 7-day supply

3 509/101.8 × 1 = 5ml per day

5 × 7 = 35ml for a 7-day supply

4 400/200 = 2 tablets per day

100/2 = 50 days

5 750/150 = 5 tablets per day

5 × 28 = 140 tablets for a 28-day supply

6 509/203.6 × 1 = 2.5ml per dose

2.5 × 2 = 5ml per day

5 × 28 = 140ml for a 28-day supply

7 3.12 × 1000 = 3120

3120/104 = 30ml

150/30 = 5 days

8 900/450 = 2 tablets per day

60/2 = 30 days

9 1g × 1000 = 1000mg

1000/200 = 5 tablets per day

5 × 28 = 140 tablets for a 28-day supply

£2.20 = 220p

220/100 = 2.2p per tablet

140 × 2.2 = 308p or £3.08

10 1.018g × 1000 = 1018mg

1018/101.8 × 1 = 10ml per day

10 × 30 = 300ml for a 30-day supply

300/150 = 2 × bottles at £5.79 = £11.58

Multiple choice questions

1 A
2 C
3 B
4 B
5 D
6 C
7 D
8 B

9 C
10 C

Case study

- Stability – why change? If Mr Khan is well maintained on his current medication it is worth exploring with him why he wishes to consider changing drugs.
- The pros and cons of changing from his current medication should be outlined to him.
- Supervised switch over should occur if a change of medication is deemed appropriate and regular review should occur during the switching period.

Chapter 11

Calculations

1. $500/200 = 2.5$ tablets per day $\times 28 = 70$ tablets for a 28-day supply

2. $150/50 = 3$ tablets for day one

    $100/50 = 2$ tablets for day two and 2 tablets for day three

    $350/50 = 7$ tablets per week

    $7 \times 4 = 28$ tablets for a 28-day supply

3. $800/2 = 400$mg per dose

    $400/200 = 2$ tablets per dose

    $2 \times 2 = 4$ tablets per day

    $4 \times 28 = 112$ tablets for a 28-day supply

4. $30/5 = 6$ tablets per day

5. $120/20 \times 1 = 6$ml per day

6. $30/10 = 3$ capsules per dose

    $3 \times 4 = 12$ capsules per day

7. 4mg $\times 1000 = 4000$micrograms

    $4000/200 \times 1 = 20$ml per dose

    $20 \times 2 = 40$ml per day

    $40 \times 14 = 560$ml for a 14-day supply

8. $16/2 = 8$mg per dose

    $8/2 = 4$ tablets per dose

    $4 \times 2 = 8$ tablets per day

$8 \times 14 = 112$ tablets for a 14-day supply

9. $10/1 \times 1 = 10$ml per dose

    $10 \times 3 = 30$ml per day

    $30 \times 5 = 150$ml for a 5-day supply

10. 20mg $+ 10$ mg $= 30$mg as a daily dose

    $30/5 = 6$ tablets for the day supply

Multiple choice questions

1. B
2. B
3. D
4. D
5. A
6. D
7. D
8. B
9. C
10. A

Case study

- Establish his current and usual drug-taking pattern.
- With Jim plan the method of medication management; is it reduction, replacement with a view to reduction or managed abstinence?
- Titration and monitoring of any pharmacological intervention will be required.
- Monitoring of withdrawal signs and pharmacological management if appropriate.
- Once daily supervised medication may be required (methadone).
- Reviews should be regular and tailored towards Jim's needs.
- Support in the form of psychosocial interventions should always be present.

Chapter 12

Multiple choice questions

1. C
2. D
3. A
4. A
5. C
6. D

7 A
8 B
9 B
10 C

Case study

- SSRIs are the first-line drug of choice based on licensing and NICE guidelines.
- Talking therapies and support must be part of Jack's treatment plan, and family therapy should be looked at as an appropriate intervention.
- Suicide prevention measures must be considered.
- Capacity to consent should be assessed using the Fraser Guidelines.

Chapter 13

Multiple choice questions

1 B
2 A
3 C
4 D
5 B
6 A
7 C
8 D
9 A
10 D

Case study

- Counselling and talking therapies are first line. Emily appears to have components of anorexia nervosa and bulimia nervosa.
- In-patient admission for specialist services may be appropriate.
- Group therapy would help Emily as she could meet and work with people in the same situation as herself.
- Feeding programme may be an issue with a body mass index of 13 and if Emily does not consent to feeding then this can be forced under the terms of the Mental Health Act. Her capacity to consent should be assessed under the Mental Capacity Act.

Index

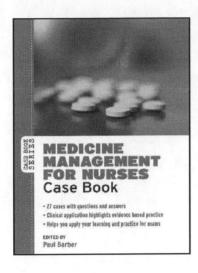

MEDICINE MANAGEMENT FOR NURSES
Case Book

Paul Barber (Ed)

9780335245758 (Paperback)
August 2013

eBook also available

This case book covers the principles and skills involved in a range of medicine management scenarios and will help nursing students integrate their knowledge of physiology, pathophysiology, pharmacology and nursing care. Including 21 case studies, each case gives readers the opportunity to learn about effective medicine management while testing their knowledge and understanding of essential drug groups.

Key features:

- The cases cover a variety of conditions helping students to learn what to do in many types of scenarios
- Includes questions, answers and other self-test features
- Aimed at nurses studying pharmacology/medicine management

www.**openup**.co.uk

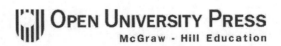

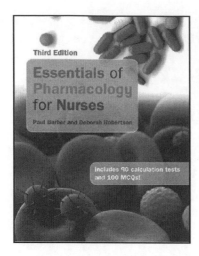

Essentials of Pharmacology for Nurses
Third Edition

Barber and Robertson

ISBN: 9780335261963 (Paperback)
eISBN: 9780335261970

2015

This ideal starter text for student nurses makes pharmacology less intimidating by focusing on the knowledge needed at pre-registration level in order to practise as a newly qualified nurse.

Praised for its helpful layout and jargon-free language, this updated edition introduces pharmacology in a friendly, informative way, without assuming previous knowledge of pharmacology or a level of confidence with maths.

This new edition has been expanded to include a new chapter introducing drug calculations and measurements as well as more detail on drugs used in chronic conditions, and on pharmacology for the older patient and other specific groups such as children, pregnant women or those with minor illness. Extra case scenarios have been added to encourage nurses to apply knowledge to a range of different people with differing needs.

The book contains:

- 90 calculations and 100 multiple choice questions to help perfect your skills and assess learning
- Clinical tip boxes linking pharmacology to the role of the nurse
- 38 patient scenarios across a range of clinical settings
- References to key clinical tests and guidelines

www.mheducation.co.uk

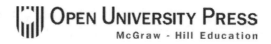

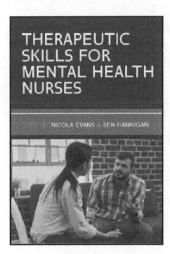

Therapeutic Skills for Mental Health Nurses

Evans and Hannigan

ISBN: 9780335264407 (Paperback)
eISBN: 9780335264414

2016

Most specialist mental health care is provided by nurses who use face-to-face helping skills with a wide range of people in a variety of contexts. This book puts therapeutic skills at the heart of the nurse's role, with one central aim: to equip you with knowledge to use in your practice, thus improving your ability to deliver care.

This book:

- Will enable you to strengthen your core therapeutic skills and broaden your knowledge to include other practical therapeutic approaches
- Collates in one place information on a range of therapeutic approaches, from person centred counselling, motivational interviewing and solution focused approaches, through to day-to-day skills of challenging unhelpful thoughts, de-escalating difficult situations, working with families, and problem solving
- Demonstrates application of theory to practice through a variety of practical examples
- Features reader activities to facilitate personal growth and learning
- Includes a chapter exploring clinical supervision and how this makes practice more effective

www.mheducation.co.uk

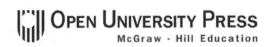
OPEN UNIVERSITY PRESS
McGraw · Hill Education

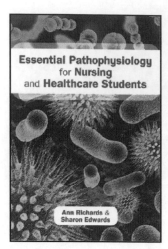

Essential Pathophysiology for Nursing and Healthcare Students

Richards and Edwards

ISBN: 9780335238323 (Paperback)
eBook: 9780335238347
2014

This is the perfect quick reference and study guide for students covering pathophysiology, disease and therapeutics as part of a nursing or other healthcare course. It clearly and simply explains the underpinning processes of disease, covering cellular physiology, genetics, fluids, electrolytes and the immune system, and the main diseases and conditions that can occur within each.

The book covers body systems including:

- Cardiovascular
- Respiratory
- Immune
- Lymphatic
- Nervous
- Digestive
- Endocrine
- Reproductive
- Renal
- Muscular-Skeletal

www.openup.co.uk

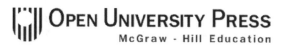

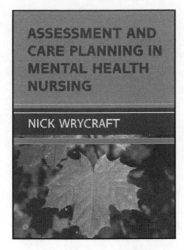

Assessment and Care Planning in Mental Health Nursing

Nick Wrycraft

ISBN: 9780335262984 (Paperback)
eBook: 9780335262991
2015

Assessment of mental health problems is a challenging area of practice that covers a range of symptoms and behaviours – and involves building a trusting relationship with the service user while also using specialist skills. Care planning involves translating information emerging from assessment to collaboratively identify goals and aspirations that are meaningful yet also realistic and personalized.

The first section of the book explores core aspects of assessment including communication skills and engaging the service user before considering risk assessment, care planning, interventions, relapse prevention and reflection. The next section will be ideal for quick reference during practice and looks at 23 different clinical behaviours that nurses will assess, under 4 categories:

Physical factors in mental health
Behavioural aspects in mental health
The role of thoughts in mental health
Feelings in mental health

www.mheducation.co.uk

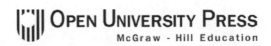